Clinical Cases in

PEDIATRICS

Clinical Cases in PEDIATRICS

R Rajamahendran
MS MRCS (Edinburgh) FMAS Dip Lap MCh (SGE)
Postgraduate in MCh Surgical Gastroenterology
Madras Medical College
Chennai, Tamil Nadu, India

Co-authors

B Parthiban MD
Assistant Professor
Department of Pediatrics
Kilpauk Medical College
Chennai, Tamil Nadu, India

K Ilayaraja MD (Pediatrics)
Assistant Professor
Department of Pediatrics
Villupuram Medical College
Villupuram, Tamil Nadu, India

Foreword
R Narayana Babu

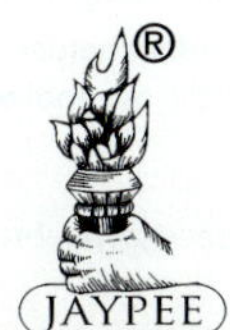

JAYPEE BROTHERS MEDICAL PUBLISHERS (P) LTD
New Delhi • London • Philadelphia • Panama

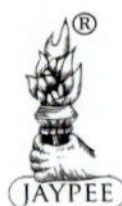

Jaypee Brothers Medical Publishers (P) Ltd

Headquarters

Jaypee Brothers Medical Publishers (P) Ltd
4838/24, Ansari Road, Daryaganj
New Delhi 110 002, India
Phone: +91-11-43574357
Fax: +91-11-43574314
Email: jaypee@jaypeebrothers.com

Overseas Offices

J.P. Medical Ltd
83 Victoria Street, London
SW1H 0HW (UK)
Phone: +44-2031708910
Fax: +02-03-0086180
Email: info@jpmedpub.com

Jaypee-Highlights Medical Publishers Inc.
City of Knowledge, Bld. 237, Clayton
Panama City, Panama
Phone: +1 507-301-0496
Fax: +1 507-301-0499
Email: cservice@jphmedical.com

Jaypee Medical Inc.
The Bourse
111 South Independence Mall East
Suite 835, Philadelphia, PA 19106, USA
Phone: +1 267-519-9789
Email: joe.rusko@jaypeebrothers.com

Jaypee Brothers Medical Publishers (P) Ltd
17/1-B Babar Road, Block-B, Shaymali
Mohammadpur, Dhaka-1207
Bangladesh
Mobile: +08801912003485
Email: jaypeedhaka@gmail.com

Jaypee Brothers Medical Publishers (P) Ltd
Bhotahity, Kathmandu, Nepal
Phone: +977-9741283608
Email: kathmandu@jaypeebrothers.com

Website: www.jaypeebrothers.com
Website: www.jaypeedigital.com

Inquiries for bulk sales may be solicited at: jaypee@jaypeebrothers.com

Clinical Cases in Pediatrics

First Edition: **2014**

ISBN: 978-93-5152-065-8

Printed at: Samrat Offset Pvt. Ltd.

Dedicated to

My dear friend

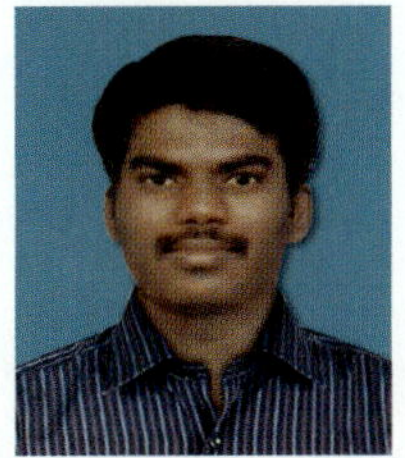

Late Dr S Karthikeyan MD (Anesthesia)

and

All the MBBS students

—R Rajamahendran

Dedicated to

My dear friend

Late Dr. J. Karthikeyan

All the ABBS students

Sajeendhanathan

FOREWORD

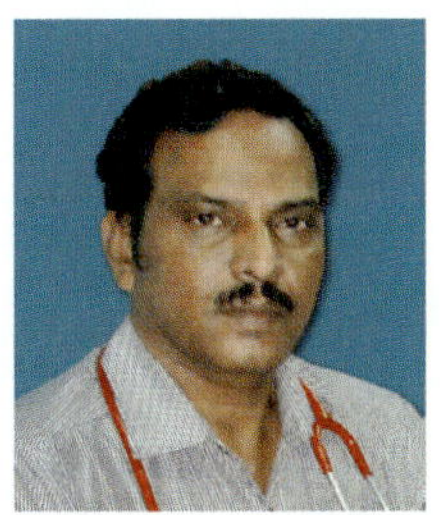

It is my immense pleasure to write the Foreword for the first edition of this book *Clinical Cases in Pediatrics* for Final MBBS students. The crisp and catchy nature of this book makes it the book of choice for Final year students. On reading the chapters, I could understand the hard efforts made by these young authors, which are enormous. They have made all the essential points we need for the MBBS students in a simplified and illustrative way so that they would not forget the concepts. I really wondered to see all the essential questions asked in the clinical examinations are explained in this short book.

The colored photographs and colored edition makes it an attractive book among the students. The materials are found updated according to the latest journals and textbooks. I wish this book will be a great success and boon to the authors. I also wish the authors to bring many similar books to the medical society.

R Narayana Babu MD DCH
Head
Department of Pediatrics
Deputy Superindent
Government Kilpauk Medical College
Chennai, Tamil Nadu, India

PREFACE

Increasing load upon the Final MBBS students on reading all the essential subjects such as Medicine, Surgery, Obstetrics, Gynecology, Orthopedics, and Pediatrics made them suffer a lot during the clinical examination. I found they tend to forget the most important points reading a lot of books during the examination. Especially pediatrics is an essential subject in the MBBS career of a student and many of them failed in their examination due to the pediatrics practical. I found there is no book available for undergraduate standard in pediatrics clinical examination methods and discussion. Hence, I decided to refine my pediatrics materials with the help of my pediatric friends Dr B Parthiban and Dr K Ilayaraja. They had helped me a lot in bringing the updated edition in spite of their busy practice.

The success of my previous clinical books for MBBS students—*Long Cases in Surgery, Short Cases in Surgery* and *Clinical Cases in Obstetrics and Gynecology* made me do this book on *Clinical Cases in Pediatrics*. The co-authors of this book tried their best in bringing the book with all essential points updating to the present standard of practice in clinical pediatrics. The chapters on Vaccines and Tuberculosis are all taken from the latest updated articles of Pediatrics in India.

The most highlighted part of this book is the crispy nature of the book, which makes it an essential book for the regular ward rounds and also the essential book for last-minute revision during the examination. "To err is human"... In spite of being written by three authors, this book may have some mistakes. Kindly send your feedbacks and point out the mistakes by mailing to me on *minnalraja@gmail.com*.

All the best to my dear students...

R Rajamahendran

ACKNOWLEDGMENTS

I have to start my acknowledgment for Shri Jitendar P Vij (Group Chairman), Mr Ankit Vij (Managing Director) and Mr Tarun Duneja (Director-Publishing) of M/s Jaypee Brothers Medical Publishers (P) Ltd, New Delhi, India, and Mr Jayanandan, Chennai Branch, who introduced me into the field of book writing and made me a renowned author. So far, I have written six books in different publications for Medicos, all the credit will go to only M/s Jaypee Brothers Medical Publishers (P) Ltd, New Delhi, India.

I have to thank Mrs Chetna Malhotra Vohra specially for giving a tremendous support in writing this book and helping me bring this book with excellent quality. I thank Mr Rajesh Sharma, for his coordination in the making of this book.

I would like to thank Prof SM Chandramohan, MCh, Head, Department of Surgical Gastroenterology; Prof D Kannan, MCh, Professor, Department of Surgical Gastroenterology; Dr Amudhan, MCh; Dr Benet Duraisamy, MCh, and Dr Prabhakaran, MCh, for their constant support during my course of postgraduation in MCh Surgical Gastroenterology.

I would like to mention the legends in pediatrics when I was doing my MBBS in 2002 in Kilpauk Medical College (KMC)—Prof R Narayana Babu (Presently in KMC) and Prof Subramaniam (Presently in Chengalpet Medical College). Their extraordinary classes made me write notes which have now transformed into a clinical book.

My special thanks to Prof Nedunchezhiyan, HOD, Dharmapuri Medical College/Chief Editor, Indian Journal of Practical Pediatrics, who created interest in academic and pediatric researches.

I would like to thank all my friends, students, and teachers, who have been supporting my books since 2007. I would like to thank my wife Dr Shanthi, and my little daughters Saadhu and Raju, for their constant motivation and support in my academic activities.

R Rajamahendran

ACKNOWLEDGMENTS

I would like to thank Dr R Rajamahendran, for giving me the chance to edit his notes and update.

I would like to express my gratitude to the many people, who made me a pediatrician and created interest in academic pediatrics.

There are many stars in my life who have brightened (and continue to brighten) my path, starting from my undergraduate teachers to the great teachers from Madras Medical College (MMC)—Institute of Child Health including the Director and Superintents such as Dr M Kannaki, Dr Jeyachandran, my professors and great teachers such as Dr P Sekar; Dr P Ramachandran; Dr S Sundari; Dr C Leema Pauline, Pediatric Neurologist; Dr Vijayasekar, Pediatric Pulmonologist; Dr Kumutha, Neonatologist; Dr Vijayakumar; Dr Rema Chandramohan, Neonatologists; Dr S Gnanasambandam, Pediatric Cardiologist; Dr Nirmala, Pediatric Gastroenterologist; Dr Padmarajan, Pediatric Nephrologist; Dr Raghunathan; Dr Subramanian; Dr Ezhilarasi; Dr Indumathi Santhanam; Dr Shanthi; Dr Devi Meenakshi, and Dr Lakshmi.

I would like to thank Pediatric Registrar of MMC—Dr Srinivasan and Dr Luke Ravi Chellaiyai.

I would like to thank my Assistant Professors—Dr Hema Chitra, Dr Sivaraman, Dr Prabahar, Dr Sumathi, Dr Kumaravel (Salem), Dr Poovazhagi, Dr Senthil Kumar, Dr Neelakandan and Dr Stalin.

My collegues need a special thanks—Dr Adal Arasan, Dr Suganya, Dr Sridevi, Dr Raja Vijaya Krishnan, Dr Thenmozhi, Dr Jeyanthi, Dr Neelakandan, Dr Suresh, Dr Giridhar, Dr Sivashankar and Dr Vinoth.

I would like to give a special thanks to the stars who are making me to learn even as Assistant Professor in Pediatrics at Government Kilpauk Medical College and Hospital such as my HOD—Dr R Narayana Babu, my Professors—Dr Jeyachandran and Dr Sathiyamorthy, who boosts me to be a good academic and clinical pediatrician.

I would like to thank my postgraduates, Compulsory Rotatory Residential Internship (CRRI), my undergraduates from KMC and MMC, who made me to update by asking a lot of questions.

I take this opportunity to thank my wife Dr Thenmozhi, MD (Derm) and my little daughter Mahalakshmi, for their constant support in my academic activities.

Last but not least, I beg forgiveness of all those who have been with me over the course of the years and whose names I have failed to mention.

B Parthiban

CONTENTS

CASE 1 Protein Energy Malnutrition

DEFINITION

It is a range of pathological conditions arising from coincident lack in varying proportions of calories and proteins, occurring frequently and commonly in infants associated with infestation, vitamin deficiency, etc. (Fig. 1.1).

CLASSIFICATION

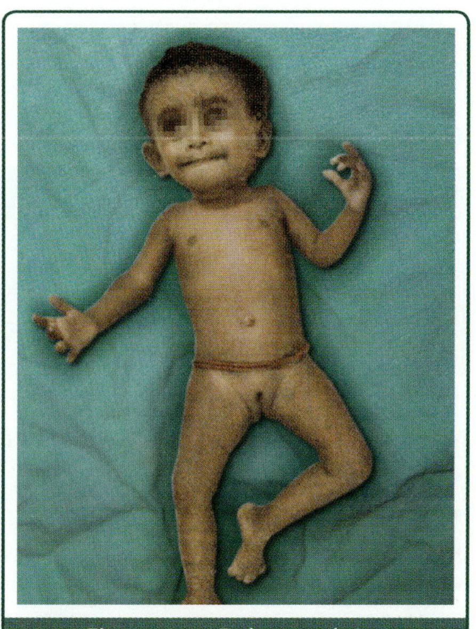

Figure 1.1: Failure to thrive

Welcome's Classification (Clinical Classification)

- Above 80% of expected weight for age: Normal
- 60–80% of expected weight without edema: Under nutrition
- 60–80% of expected weight with edema: Kwashiorkor
- <60% of expected weight without edema: Marasmus
- <60% of expected weight with edema: Marasmic-kwashiorkor.

Gomez Classification (International)

- >90%: Normal
  - Grade I—90–75% of expected weight for age
  - Grade II—79–60% of expected weight for age
  - Grade III—<60% of expected weight for age.

IAP Classification (Indian)

- Grade I—80–70% of expected weight for age
- Grade II—70–60% of expected weight for age
- Grade III—60–50% of expected weight for age
- Grade IV—<50% of expected weight for age
- Add (K) to presence of edema.

Jellife's Classification (Based on Weight)

- Normal—>90%
  - Grade I—80–90%
  - Grade II—70–79%
  - Grade III—60–69%
  - Grade IV—<60%.

Waterlow's Classification

Weight/height	*Height/age*	*Labs*
≥80%	≥90% ≤90%	Normal Stunted
≤80%	≥90% ≤ 90%	Wasted Wasted and stunted

Arnold's Classification

	MAC (cm)
a. Normal:	≥13.5
b. Mild–moderate:	12.5–13.4
c. Severe:	≤12.4

Gopalan's Classification

Types of PEM	*Weight/age*	*Height/age*	*Weight/height*
Acute PEM	Decreased	Equivalent	Decreased
Chronic PEM	Decreased	Decreased	Equivalent
Chronic active	Decreased	Decreased	Decreased

You must ask the history of following in PEM case without fail:

- H/O Measles
- H/O Worms in stool
- H/O Tuberculosis contact
- H/O Recurrent UTI
- H/O Recurrent respiratory tract infection
- H/O Ear discharge
- H/O Any surgeries
- H/O Pica (eating stones, soil, waste papers, chalk)
  - Iron deficiency
  - lead poisoning anemia
  - Perverted habit of eating
- H/O Regurgitation (cleft palate)
- H/O Vomiting (GERD) and regurgitation
- H/O Lactose intolerance/malabsorption
  - A: Abdomen distension
  - B: Borborygmi (abnormal bowel sounds)
  - C: Colicky abdomen pain
  - D: Diarrhea
  - E: Excoriation (perianal)
  - F: Flatus
- H/O: Renal cause/cardiac cause of edema.

ANTENATAL HISTORY

- Remember **3 I**'s
  - **I**nfection
  - **I**rradiation
  - **I**ngestion of drugs
- Booked/unbooked
- Immunization, number of antenatal visits, failure to gain weight, preeclampsia, preterm/IUGR/hypoxia
- Any illness—hospitalization, drug intake, irradiation
- Iron/folic acid tablets given
- H/O Diet
- Working mother
- Mental stress
- Age of mother during pregnancy.

NATAL HISTORY

- NFTD (normal full term delivery)/preterm/cesarean
- Forceps
- Domiciliary/hospital
- Cried immediately/birth weight
- Breastfeed given after how many hours.

POSTNATAL HISTORY (30 DAYS)

- Any infection
- Any H/O neonatal intensive care unit (NICU) admission
- Breastfeeding adequate/duration/adequate means (8–10 feeds/day)
- H/O Bottle-feeding
- H/O Prelacteal feeds
- H/O Weaning (early or late)—complementary feeding habit
  - H/O Loss of appetite
  - H/O Loss of weight.

DEVELOPMENTAL HISTORY

- Milestones
  - Motor
  - Fine motor
  - Social adaptation
  - Language
- Tell the milestone of which age the child belongs to
  - Milestones: Described separately.

DIET HISTORY

- Breastfed—how long/times/day/colostrum milk given or not?
- Bottle-fed—what milk/diluted or not/how much?
- How much calories the baby is taking?
- Expected calories?
- Deficit chart/requirement chart.

FAMILY HISTORY/SOCIAL HISTORY

- Consanguineous babies—low birth weight is more
- Socioeconomic status
- Number of siblings—spacing (normal—3 years)
- Occupation of parents
- Per capita income
- H/O Any illness in family
- Area: Rural/urban
- Slum/industrialized zone
- Type of home: Tiles, rooms, hut
- Drinking water source
- Type of latrine
- Waste disposal.

Kuppuswamy Scoring

- Based on family income, education and occupation
- Symbols:

-	Non-consanguineous marriage
=	Consanguineous marriage
➚	This baby concerned
Ø	Dead baby—cause of death
!	Aborted

- Pedigree chart:

Model Pedigree chart

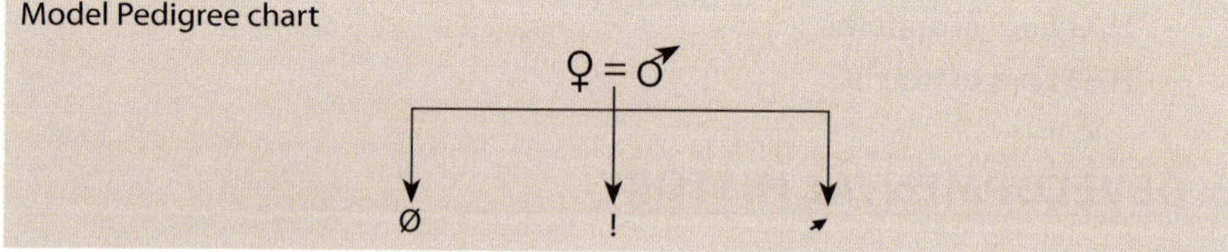

- Birth spacing
- Family planning.

IMMUNIZATION HISTORY

- 9 and 15 months: 2 doses of measles
- 5 years: Again DPT
- At 10 years: Tetanus toxoid should be given (most of them, not aware).

CONTACT HISTORY

- Tuberculosis (no H/O contact with open case of TB).

Classification of Consanguinity

Social classification	*Genetic classification*
1st degree: Marrying brothers and sisters	1st degree: Sharing 50–50% genes
2nd degree: Maternal uncles	2nd degree: Sharing 75% and 25% genes
3rd degree: Cousins and distant relatives	3rd degree: No sharing

GENERAL EXAMINATION

- Conscious, cooperative, oriented
- Attitude, look
- Appearance: Irritable/dull/mental apathy/lethargic
  - Old man or monkey appearance—marasmus
  - Moon face—kwashiorkor
  - Not interested in surroundings
- Generalized wasting
- Skin folds
- Anemia, jaundice, clubbing, lymphadenopathy and cyanosis
- Pedal edema
- Fontanelles.

Anterior fontanelle	*Posterior fontanelle*
Normal size = 2.5 × 2.5 cm (across borders) Normal closure—9–18 months	Closes by 2–4 months
Delayed closure: • Rickets • Hypothyroidism • Hydrocephalus • Down syndrome • Achondroplasia • Mucopolysaccharidosis Early closure: • Craniosynostosis • Primary microcephaly	

HEAD TO FOOT EXAMINATION

Mental State

- Apathy: Kwashiorkor (resents examination)
- Irritable: Marasmus (not allowing the examination and becomes angry)
- Generalized wasting.

Hair

- Space
- Color
- Easy pluckability
- Flag sign
- Alopecia
- Fungal infection.

Hair change is because of
- Decreased tyrosine
- Decreased melanin
- Decreased copper
- Decreased cysteine

Anterior Fontanelle

- Wide open, depressed and delayed closure in PEM
- Bulging anterior fontanelle: Increased intracranial tension, while crying (physiological).

Head Circumference

Eyes

- Anemia
- Sunken eyes
- Vitamin A deficiency .

Ear

Discharge

Nose

Rhinitis

Mouth

- Angular stomatitis
- Ulcer, cheilosis
- Anemia, glossitis
- Candidal infection
- Dental caries, tonsil, oral thrush
- Cleft lip and palate (more prone for regurgitation)
- No of teeth (delayed eruption in PEM).

Permanent teeth
- 1st molar—6 years
- Central and lateral—6–8 years
- Central < premolar—9–12 years
- Second molar—12 years
- 3rd molar—18 years

Neck

- Lymphadenopathy—axillary and cervical.

Skin Changes

(It is because of decreased—tyrosine/melanin)

- Dry scaly (decreased proline/hydroxyproline)
- Ulcer in flexors
- Gangrenous lesions
- Skin turgor—loss of elasticity
- Purpuric spots—gram negative sepsis
- Crazy pavement appearance.

Abdominal Distension (Hypoproteinemia)

- Hepatosplenomegaly
- Free fluid
- Umbilical hernia.

Foot

Edema

Anal Excoriation

(In diarrhea cases) rectal prolapse

1. Perianal excoriation
2. Beaver diarrhea
3. Loss of perirectal pad of fat, due to PEM.

Other Vitamin Deficiencies

Rickets

Vitals

- Temp: Hypothermia
- BP
- Pulse: Rapid thready/tachy or bradycardia
- Respiratory rate.

Temperature:
Normal temperature: 36.5–37.5°C
<5 years: Groin, axilla or rectal temperature used
>5 years: Oral temperature
Remember;
Axilla and groin—0.5°C lower than oral
Rectal—0.5°C greater than oral

- Hyperpyrexia means temperature >37°C

Normal respiratory rate:
Newborn = 40/min
1 year = 30/min
5 years = 20/min
10 years = 18/min

Normal BP (IAP)
Newborn—65/45 mm Hg
1 year—75/50 mm Hg
3 years—90/60 mm Hg
8 years—95/65 mm Hg
10 years—100/70 mm Hg

BP—flash method:
- Always measure BP in both upper limbs and lower limbs to R/O coarctation of aorta
- Normally: In upper limbs, BP is 10 mm Hg lesser than lower limb

ANTHROPOMETRY

Always write the expected:
1. Weight
2. Height
3. Head circumference
4. Mid-arm circumference
5. Chest circumference.

Weight of Baby

- Normal at birth: 2.8 kg
  - Spring balance
  - Infant weighing scale
  - Salter weighing scale
  - Beam scale
- Up to 3 months: Increases at 30–50 g/day

3 months – 1 year: $\frac{\text{Age in months} + 9}{2}$

1 – 6 years: (Age in years x 2) + 8

7 – 12 years: $\frac{(\text{Age in years x } 7) - 5}{2}$

- At 5 months—Doubles
- At 1 years—Triples
- At 2 years—4 times
- At 3 years—5 times
- At 5 years—6 times
- At 10 years—10 times
  - 2 years—12 kg
  - Add 2 kg/year thereafter.

Newborn Weight Status

- New born loses up to 10% of body weight in 1 week
- Regains lost weight by 10 days
- 25–30 g/day (next 3 months)
- 400 g/month

Height

- Vertical scale
- Measuring rod
- Stadiometer.

IAP

Age	*Height (in cm)*
At birth	50 cm
½ year	62 cm
1 year	75 cm
2 years	87.5 cm
3–5 years	6–8 cm/year
>5 years	5 cm/year

Average height at birth: 50 cm

- Height increases by 3 cm/month =1st 3 months
- Height increases by 2 cm/month = 2nd 3 months
- Height increases by 1.5cm/month = up to 3 next 3 months
- Height increases by 1 cm/month = upto 2 years

- At 1 year: 75 cm
- 2 years: 87 cm

Weech's formula for height	
Age	*Height (in cm)*
At birth	50 cm
At 1 year	75 cm
2–12 years	(Age in years x 6) + 77

- Length measured by infant meter until the child is ambulant
  - $$\text{Growth Velocity} = \frac{\text{Initial height (in cm)} - \text{height at next measurement}}{\text{Time period between 2 measures}}$$
  - $$\text{Growth Index} = \frac{\text{Actual growth velocity}}{\text{Expected growth velocity}} \times 100$$
    (N: 93–105% of normal)

Age	Weight	Height	Head circumference	Chest circumference	Mid-arm circumference
Birth	2.8 kg	50 cm	33 cm	32 cm	13.5 cm
I year	Triples	76 cm	45 cm	45 cm	13.5 cm

Head Circumference (HC)

- At birth = 32–35 cm (average: 35 cm)
- 1 years = 45 cm
- 2 years = 48 cm
- 12 years = 52 cm
- 18 years = 55 cm
- 1–6 months: 1–1.2 cm/month increase
- 2nd 6 months: 0.5 cm/month increase
  - >2SD = Macrocephaly
  - < 3SD = Microcephaly

Each SD = 5% of particular expected head circumference

- Fix the prominence of occiput cross over the tape and see (Take 3 times).

Chest Circumference (Measured at the Level of Nipples)

At birth, 3 cm less than head circumference

At 1 year = Both are equal

After that, chest circumference (CC) increases.

- Baby born of diabetic mother: Chest circumference > head circumference
- In malnutrition: Chest circumference < head circumference (even after 1 and a half years)

Mid-arm Circumference (MAC)

(To direct malnutrition in 1–4 years of age)

1. Tape method: Midpoint between acromion and olecranon
2. Shakir's tape: Green color: 13–16 cm = well nourished
   Yellow color: 12.5–13.5 cm = Mild-moderate
   Red color: <12.5 cm = Malnourished
   Normal is 13.5–16.5 cm for 1–4 years
   (It is constant because the subcutaneous tissue and fat replaced by muscles)
3. Logerson's Bangle test:
   Inner diameter of bangle is 4 cm
   If it easily passes and comes out of their elbow = Malnourished
4. Quack stick Method:
   For each height, a corresponding mid-arm circumference can be measured
5. Kanawati's index:
   (To detect PEM between 4 months to 4 years)

$\frac{MAC}{HC}$	
>0.32	Normal
0.26–0.32	Moderate
<0.25	Severe

Systemic Examination

1. **CVS:** Anemia and hyperdynamic in circulation, signs of heart failure, venous hum, tachycardia.
2. **RS:** Bronchopneumonia, pneumonitis, pyothorax.
3. **CNS:** Stunting, developmental delay, apathetic, irritable and mental retardation.
4. **Abdomen:** Hepatosplenomegaly.

What type of Liver is there in Kwashiorkor?

- Rounded lower margin
- Soft consistency

DIAGNOSIS
Protein energy malnutrition grade 4 according to IAP, marasmic kwashiorkor precipitated by diarrhea, lower respiratory tract infection/associated with low socioeconomic status, ignorance, illiteracy and habits

INVESTIGATIONS

1. Blood: Complete hemogram
   TC/DC/ESR/PS
2. Urine analysis: Associated UTI
   Albumin
   Deposits
   E/s
3. Motion examination: Ova/cysts/occult blood
4. X-ray chest/Mantoux: R/O TB
5. Blood C/S (septicemia)
6. Serum A:G ratio and total proteins [Normal Sr Albumin: 3.5–5 g/dL, Sr Globulin: 2–3.5 g/dL]
7. Serum electrolytes and blood sugar
8. Stool pH (acidic) and Benedict's solution (sugar)—positive in lactose intolerance
9. Blood cholesterol
10. Serum iron/copper

Diagnosis of lactose intolerance: Stool pH <5.5 for 2 occasions, after giving mild diet.

MANAGEMENT

1. Resuscitation: Treatment of emergencies and complications
2. Rehabilitation: Protein/carbohydrates
3. Supportive

Mc LAREN'S SCORING:

Edema-3
Dermatosis-2
Edema and dermatosis -6
Hepatomegaly-1
Skin changes-1
Hair changes-1

Serum albumin

- < 1 mg: 7
- < 3.5 mg: 2

Inference:

- Greater than 7= marasmus
- 5–7 is kwashiorkor

Viva: What are the age-independent criteria for assessment of PEM?

1. Weight for height:

$$\frac{\text{Weight of the child (observed)}}{\text{Weight corresponding for height of the child (expected)}} \times 100$$

<90% : PEM
>90% : Normal
>120–130%: Obesity

2. Rao index = $\frac{\text{Wt [kg]}}{\text{Ht [cm]}^2} \times 100$

3. Dugdale index: $\frac{\text{Wt [kg]}}{\text{Ht [cm] 1.6}} \times 100$ H: 0.88 – 0.97
<0.79—severe malnutrition

4. Enderberg's Index
5. Mid-arm circumference
6. Skin fold thickness:

Tricep skinfold thickness: Harpenden skin caliper

Age	Male in mm	Female in mm
5	6.1 + 2.54	9.56 + 1.87
10	9.5 + 3.69	11.5 + 3.58
15	9.03 + 3.07	14.08 + 4.47

<60% : Severe Malnutrition
60–80% : Moderate
80–90% : Mild
80–100% : Normal

Viva: What is McLaren's classification:

- Measure the height
- Compare with height at that age
  - Below 80% : Dwarf
  - 80–93% : Short
  - 93–105% : Normal
- Other H/A based classification:
  - Waterlow: Ht/Age >95% normal
  - Marginal: 90–95%
  - Moderate: 85–90%
  - Severe: 85% below

WHO Classification for Undernutrition

Age	*Moderate nutrition*	*Severe undernutrition*
Symmetrical edema	absent	Yes[xx]
Weight for height (measure of wasting)	SD score −2 to −3 (70–79% expected)	SD score <−3 (< 70% of expected)
Height for age (measure of stunting)	SD score −2 to −3 (85–89% expected)	SD score <−3 (<85% of expected)

xx-*Includes marasmic kwashiorkor and kwashiorkor*

$$\textbf{SD Score} = \frac{\text{Observed value} - \text{Expected value}}{\text{SD of reference population}} \quad \text{(SD = standard deviation)}$$

OTHER ANTHROPOMETRIC INDICES

Upper Segment/ Lower Segment Ratio

- At Birth: 1.8/1
- 3–4 years: 1.3/1
- 9 years: 1/1
- 18 years: 0.9/1

Rao's Body Mass Index

$$\frac{\text{Weight}}{\text{Height}^2} \times 100$$

- Weight in kg and height in meter square

This remains constant upto 5 years

- Values less than <18 indicates malnutrition
  - >30: Obese
  - 25–30: Overweight
  - 18–25: Normal
  - <18: Undernutrition

Quetelet Index

(Similar to Body Mass Index except Ht in cm (with no square)

$$\frac{\text{Wt (kg)}}{\text{Ht (cm)}}$$

- Normal value: 0.14–0.16
- <0.14 = Gross malnutrition

Enderberg's Index

Enderberg Index (Logarithm of Dugdale)

C = log(Wt) – 1.6 log(Ht)

- Normal value of C = 0.40
- Age independent upto = 13 years

Dugdale's Index

$$\frac{\text{Weight in kg}}{(\text{Height in cm})^{1.6}} \times 100$$

- Normal Value: 0.88–0.97
- <0.79: Severely malnourished

Quack Stick Method

- Weight measuring rod calibrated in MAC rather than height
- Values of 80% MAC for height are marked on stick
- If a child is taller than his MAC = Malnourished.

Kanawati's Index

$\frac{MAC}{HC}$	
> 0.32	Normal
0.28–0.32	Mild undernutrition
0.25–0.28	Moderate undernutrition
< 0.25	Severe undernutrition

Ponderal Index

$$\textbf{Ponderal Index} = \frac{\text{Weight in (kg)}}{\sqrt[3]{\text{Ht (cm)}}} \times 100$$

- Used in newborn
  - >2: Symmetrical IUGR
  - <2: Asymmetrical IUGR

Stem Stature Index (Crown Rump Length Index)

Height as a percentage of standing height

- At birth—67%
- 1 year—64%
- 20 years—50%

(CRL—crown to ischial tuberosity)

Skin Fold Thickness (Harpenden Skin Calipers)

- Triceps: Skin fold is picked up in the posterior surface of triceps muscle
- Subscapular: Skin is picked immediately below inferior angle of scapula
- Biceps: Over the belly of biceps.

Arm Span

Distance between tips of middle fingers with both arm held wide open, i.e. spread a part.

- Young children: 1–2 cm < height
- At 10 years: Arm span = height
- After 10 years: Arm span (1–2 cm) > height.

MARASMUS (FIG. 1.2)

Etiology

Primary Causes

- Poor diet
- Poor hygiene
- Poor education
- Dietary origin: Inadequate diet
- Infections: Gastroenteritis
- Poor socioeconomic group—maternal malnutrition
- Lack of parents education.

Secondary Causes

1. Age: Common in infants than in old children
2. Chronic vomiting:
   - Congenital hypertrophic pyloric stenosis

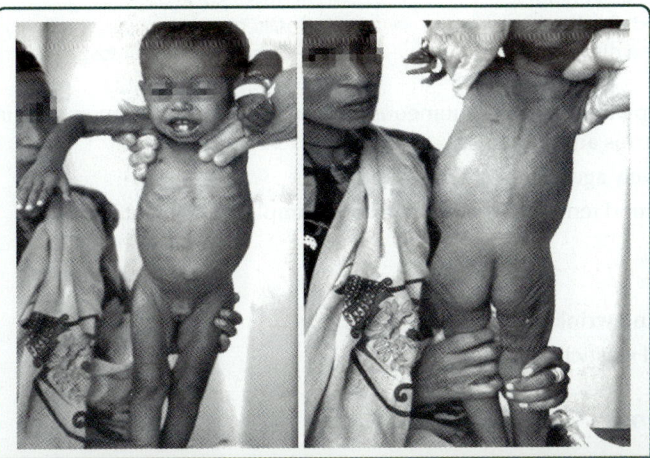

Figure 1.2: Loss of weight; more than 50% of expected weight/age with marked wasting of muscle subcutaneous fat

- Achalasia cardia
- Diaphragmatic hernia

3. Repeated diarrhea
4. Chronic infections: Congenital syphilis, empyema thoracis, tuberculosis and URI
5. Congenital diseases:
   - Cleft palate
   - Micrognathia
   - Hydrocephalus
   - Congenital penal disorders
   - Hirschsprung's disease (megacolon)
6. Organic disorders:
   - Brain, heart, kidney
   - Celiac disease
   - Mucoviscidosis
7. Metabolic disorder:
   - Infantile renal actions
   - Galactosemia
   - Diabetes.

Classification

1. Grade I : Loss of fat in axilla and groin.
2. Grade II: Loss of fat in axilla and groin and even the abdomen, and gluteal.
3. Grade III: 1 and 2 in addition, even in chest and spine.
4. Grade IV: Buccal pad of fat is lost.

Viva: Why the buccal pad of fat remains until end?

- Because it contains more of saturated fatty acids.

Clinical Feature

M- Muscle wasting	**S-** Skin inelastic
A- Active in beginning	**M-** Moniliasis
R- Repeated diarrhea	**O-** Old man face
A- Abdomen disorders	**S-** Subcutaneous fat lost

O/E : Complete loss of subcutaneous fat from buttocks, abdomen, medial aspect of thigh and arms and even face.

- Primitively aged look (old man look)
- Cheeks and temples are hollow, due to complete loss of fat.

Skin

- Loose and wrinkled
- Loses of elasticity purpura.

Abdomen

- Distended/Scaphoid
- Intestinal peristalsis visible (VIP).

Muscles

- Grossly wasted.

CNS

- Irritable and cry loudly (since, he is hungry)
- Later when infection sets in becomes apathetic and less active
  - Constipation (early)
  - Recurrent
  - Dehydration + (difficult to identity)
  - Severe electrolyte imbalance—neurologic signs and convulsions.

Others

- Moniliasis
- Cancrum oris
- Bronchopneumonia.

Biochemical Changes

- Plasma proteins are not severely reduced
- BMR increased
- Plasma volume increased.

Pathological Changes

- Weight of many organs decreases: Spleen, liver, gonads
  - Liver does not show fatty vacuolation
  - Pancreatic acini appear normal.

Diagnosis

1. Diet history
2. Physical: Congenital disorders: R/O achalasia cardia
   Infections (GIT, renal, lungs)
3. Investigations: R/O TB
   X-rays for evidence of any infections
   Pyloric stenosis
   Cardiac malformation.

Management

- Diet to be gradually increased for 2–3 weeks
- To start with high protein/thickened milk given by gavage feeding
- Treat infections
- Surgical correction (pyloric stenosis, cleft palate, diaphragmatic hernia, megacolon)
- Balanced diet and drugs.

Prognosis

Recovery begins after a latent period of 2–4 weeks.

KWASHIORKOR (FIG. 1.3)

Term coined by Dr Cicely Williams

Classical Features

- Triad of
  - Edema
  - Lethargy
  - Growth failure
- Kwashiorkor means red hair boy
- Syndrome of changeling

Overall incidence of PEM: 3–10% in India
(With marasmus and kwashiorkor)

Incidence

- South India (most common)
- 1–2% of preschool children in India
- Suffer from kwashiorkor

Age

Common: 1–3 years age

Etiology

Poverty

- Poor socioeconomic factors
- Unable to get animal-protein foods
- Non-availability of protein-rich foods
  - **Poverty index:** Expressed in term of deficient caloric intake. 70% Indians are below poverty line.

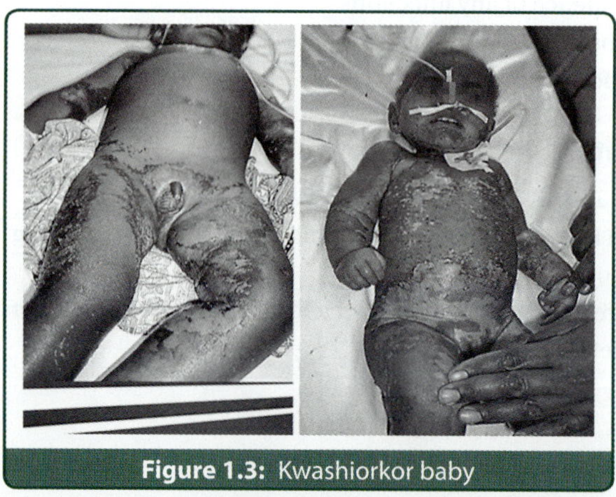

Figure 1.3: Kwashiorkor baby

Faulty Feeding Habits

- Ignorance
- Superstitions
- Prejudices.

Kwashiorkor is usually due to sudden causes:

- Infections
- Disposed child
- Increased demand
- Seasonal.

Prolonged Breastfeeding

- It actually protects against PEM (Protein energy malnutrition)
- Prolonged breastfeeding leads to 'addiction' and 'relativism' develops against food.

Infections and Infestations

- **Healthy child → Infection → Undernutrition → PEM**

If infection and undernutrition are not corrected simultaneously, the cycle cannot be broken.

- H/O
  - Recurrent diarrhea
  - Dysentery
  - Warm infestations
  - Measles
  - Tuberculosis
  - Respiratory infections

Sudden Loss of Protein

When a breastfed infant is suddenly stopped from breastfeeding, the quantity required is lost. As the factors in utero displaces this child, this condition is known as 'Deposed Child' or 'Displaced Child Syndrome'.

Sudden Demand

Already undernourished child gets a sudden lines, e.g. measles needs extra protein.

Seasonal Incidence

Peak in India: July/August (infective diarrheal period)

Size of Family

>4 or 5 children: Incidence increased by 2 or 3 times.

Clinical Profile

Apathy

- Gradual loss of interest and activity
- Children first becomes peevish
- Degree of unresponsiveness is directly proportional to severity .

Diarrhea

- 2/3 have looseness of stool
- Steatorrhea in some cases.

Malabsorption Syndrome

- Acquired intolerance to lactose may result in diarrhea—improve by excluding carbohydrate in diet
- Magnesium deficiency may also be responsible for chronic diarrhea.

Edema

- Pitting type
- Marks the muscle coating (if present)
- Ascites is rare
- Both physiochemical and hormonal factors play a part in pathogenesis.

Gopalan Postulate: Imperfect deactivation of ADH of posterior pituitary by damaged liver.

- No relation between edema and albumin.

Muscle Wasting Nutritional Hypotonia

- Weakness
- Flabbiness
- Hypotonic

O/E: Diminution or complete absence of DTR (deep tendon reflex); clinical picture is suggestive of damage to anterior horn cells, though there is no weakness.

Skin Changes

40–60% of florid kwashiorkor cases exhibits skin changes

1. **Dry and Scaly Skin:**
   - Appears cracked over large areas of trunk and limbs
   - "Mosaic pattern"
2. **Crazy-pavement dermatosis:**
   - Seen in 50% cases
   - 'Jet black patches' appear over certain localized areas, especially the pressure sites and flexures.

     This peeling plaques of dormitory resemble peeling of paint 'Flaky Paint Dermatosis'

     Discoloration is red or purple but not black.
3. **Deep fissures (ulcers)**
   - Elbows, groins, knees, behind ears
4. **Multiple puncture pinkish areas:**
   - Over the legs due to perifollicular hemorrhage(petechia/ecchymosis)
5. **Angular stomatitis**
   - Riboflavin deficiency
6. **Gangrenous dermatitis:**
   - If complicated: by severe pyogenic skin infection
   - Note **phrynoderma: Look for vitamin A-deficiency, essential fatty acid deficiency. Deficiency of tyrosine, melanin and copper.**

Hair Changes

- Scanty
- Lusterless
- Brownish/less black in Indians.

Discoloration of hair: (Dyschromotrichia) should be looked after rubbing the oil applied to hair

- **Flag sign: Patients who have been cured show segmental discoloration of hair, corresponding to period of deprivation**
- Eye lashes/brows may also be affected
- Record hair growth (N-8 mm/month)

Hepatomegaly

- 'Fatty infiltration' of liver normal consistency.

Facies

- Cheeks appear full
  (Due to hydration of cells of buccal fat)
- Moon face **(baggy cheeks of trawell)**

Avitaminosis

- 1/3 cases vitamin A deficiency
- 53% angular stomatitis
- Manifestations of Rickets (vit D deficiency) and
  - Scurvy (vit C deficiency) are extremely rare in these babies because of delayed osseous growth.

Anemia: Moderate (7–11 g)

- Normochromic/normoblastic
- 1/3rd have megaloblastc bone marrow

Other hematological features:

- Decreased white cell response to infection
- Hypoplastic bone marrow
- Abnormalities of clotting

Growth Failure

- Underweight in spite of edema
- Height is less affected than weight
- Bone growth decreased
- Severe malnutrition in early part of life results in permanent and irreversible growth retardation.

Sugar Babies: The failure of growth is not obvious in those who are previously well-nourished, they recover promptly on a high protein diet.

Psychomotor Changes

Show permanent physical and mental retardation.

Cardiovascular System

- Heart X-ray: Small head
- During recovery: Heart size increases (indicating poor cardiac reserve)
- Severe kwashiorkor: Poor peripheral circulation
  - Cyanosis
  - Hypotension
  - Feeble pulse
- Tachycardia and often bradycardia
- Evidence of CCF (after infusions)
- Arrhythmias (after digitalis) (due to decreased k+/mg++)

Biochemical Changes

1. **Serum protein**
   - Invariably reduced
   - Serum albumin <1.5 g
   - Alpha 1, 2 globulin: Increased
   - Beta globulin: Decreased
   - Gamma globulin: Increased

Normal:
Serum albumin: 4–5.3 g/dL
Serum globulin: 2–3.5 g/dL
A:G ratio is reversed in PEM (Increased globulin and decreased albumin)

2. Amino acids:
   - Decrease in essential amino acids
   - Decreased amino nitrogen/total nitrogen
   - Aminoaciduria +

   HOP index: Hydroxyproline index: Increased (Normal: 4.7)

   Marasmus: This ratio is decreased.

   Hydroxyproline is an important constituent of collagen.
3. Blood Cholesterol: Low and reduced to 90–120 mg%
4. Pancreatic enzymes: Trypsin, lipase and amylase decreased.
5. Serum iron/copper: Decreased (due to reduced transferrin).
6. Water and electrolytes: Disturbed, hypomagnesemia, phosphorous depletion.

Pathological Changes

Liver

- Fat accumulates first at periphery
- Fat vacuolation is reversible and regresses with treatment
- Necrosis never occurs
- Fibrosis 2% present is minimal
- Never progresses to cirrhosis usually.

Pancreas

- Small with severe atrophy of acinar cells with severe atrophy of cells
- Islets are normal.

Gastrointestinal Tract

- Atrophic changes occur in stomach
- Intestinal villi show marked atrophy.

Heart

- Flabby, pale and thin with enlarged ventricular chambers
- Histology—atrophy of muscle fibers, fatty degeneration, mural thrombi in ventricles.

Treatment

There are 10 essential steps in two phases:

- Initial stabilization phase
- Longer rehabilitation phase

Initial stabilization phase upto 7 days
Rehabilitation phase from 2–6 weeks

The 10 essential steps are:

1. Hypoglycemia correction
2. Hypothermia correction
3. Dehydration correction
4. Electrolyte correction
5. Infection control
6. Micronutrients without iron in early phase and with iron in late phase
7. Initiate feeding
8. Catch up growth
9. Sensory stimulation
10. Prepare for follow up

1. **Protein: 4 g/kg body weight**

   Study of children with PEM showed, they need:
   - 2 g milk protein/kg
   - 150 cal/kg/day

   5–6 g/kg needed in infections.
2. **Calories: 120–150 cal/kg/day**

   Severely affected: Require IV infusion of proteins and calories

   Glucose + electrolytes: Infused with great care as not to cardiac load

   Therefore, use diuretics to prevent edema with cardiac failure.
3. **Control of infections: Diarrhea by fluid therapy**
4. **Correction of metabolic derangements:**
   I. Hypoglycemia: IV infusion 10% (cure 5–10 mg) (kg)
   II. Hypokalemia: Potassium 5 Eq/kg
   III. Hypothermia: Electric bulbs, wrapping with two fold cloth

IV. Magnesium deficiency: Parenteral magnesium sulfate for 3–7days
V. Anemia: Blood transfusion. Iron and other hematinics (Folic acid/B_{12})
VI. Vit A def: IM 50,000 to 1,00,000 Units

Course/Prognosis

Overall Mortality 7–20%

- Most deaths occur without warning on 1–3 days of the admission.

Cause of Death

- 3H
  - **H**ypothermia
  - **H**ypoglycemia
  - **H**eart failure

Prevention

- N- Nutrition
- I- Immunization
- M- Medical care
- F- Family health
- E- Education on nutrition and health
- S- Stimulation and development

Nutritional Recovery Syndrome (NRS)

The symptoms of NRS appear when child starts to recover after a latent period of 2–4 weeks. This is due to treatment with high quality of proteins mechanism not known.

- C/F – Excessive appetite
  - Distension of abdomen
  - Reappearance of mild edema
  - Shining skin over legs
- O/E – Liver enlarged
  - Moon facies
  - Rapid weight gain
  - Apathetic child starts smiling
  - Weight gain = 2–3 kg/week
- Appetite is voracious and mothers hesitate to feed for fear of diarrhea.

Investigations

- BP increases
- 17-ketosteroid in urine increased

This syndrome is thought to be due to

1. Recovering function of adrenals
2. Increase in size and increased steroid secretion

Viva Questions from PEM

- Why there is mental retardation in kwashiorkor?
  - Hypoalbuminemia
  - Hypoglycemia—decreased supply to brain of nutrients leading to MR

- What are the causes of hepatomegaly in kwashiorkor?
  - CCF
  - Fatty liver
  - Infections
  - Tuberculosis

  If ascites is present—think of other complication
- Why there is a distended abdomen in PEM?
  - Hypokalemia → Hypotonia
- Zinc deficiency manifests as acrodermatitis enterpathica (Necklace dermatitis)
- What is the 1st sign of recovery?
  - Child becomes active and starts to eat well
- What are the early features of vitamin A deficiency? (Fig. 1.4)

  Early sign—loss of guttural pigmentation

  Early symptom—night blindness.

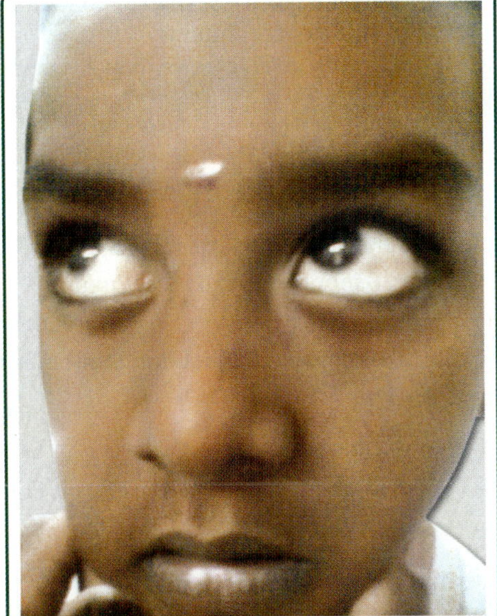

Figure 1.4: Bitot's spot—vitamin A deficiency

1. What is Pica?

   Craving for non-edible substance

   Complications:
   - Calculi
   - Lead poisoning
   - Worm infestations
   - Anemia
   - Stone formation
   - Suffocation.
2. What is the extra requirement in antenatal period?

   +14 g protein
   +300 kcal energy
3. What is the supplement in mid-day meal program?

   1/3 calories and 1/3 protein requirement of that child.
4. What do you infer from?

   Instable child -Depletion of calories more

   Lethargic child - Depletion of proteins more
5. Endocrine causes of PEM?

   Diabetes mellitus and insipidus.
6. Pseudoparalysis is seen in:
   - Congenital syphilis
   - Osteomyelitis
   - Scurvy
   - Septic arthritis
7. Vit A supplementation program:

   Between: 6 months–3 years

- Why not given less than 6 months? Breast milk contains 53 microgram which is sufficient for infants.
- Why not given greater than 2 years? Child starts taking food of adult value.

Vit A dose: <6 months—50,000 IU
6 months–1 year—1 lakh IU
1–5 years—2 lakh IU

8. What is the prophylaxis for vit A?

Every 6 months: 2 lakh IU of Vitamin A

Mild vit. A deficiency: (c/o: Bitot's spot, night blindness)	20,000 IU/day for 10 days or 2 lac IU as a single dose
Severe form: (c/o: keratomalacia corneal xerosis)	Parenteral vit supplement: 1 lakh IU 1st day 1 lakh IU 2nd day 2 lakh IU (oral) 14 days later

9. **WHO classification:**

XN: Night Blindness
X1A: Conjunctival xerosis
1B : Bitots spot (Fig. 1.5)
X2: Corneal xerosis
X3A: Corneal ulceration (cornea < 1/3 surface)
X3B: Keratomalacia (cornea >1/3 surface)
XF: Xerophthalmic fundus
XS: Corneal scars

10. What is the contraindication for ORS?
    - Persistent vomiting in an unconscious child.

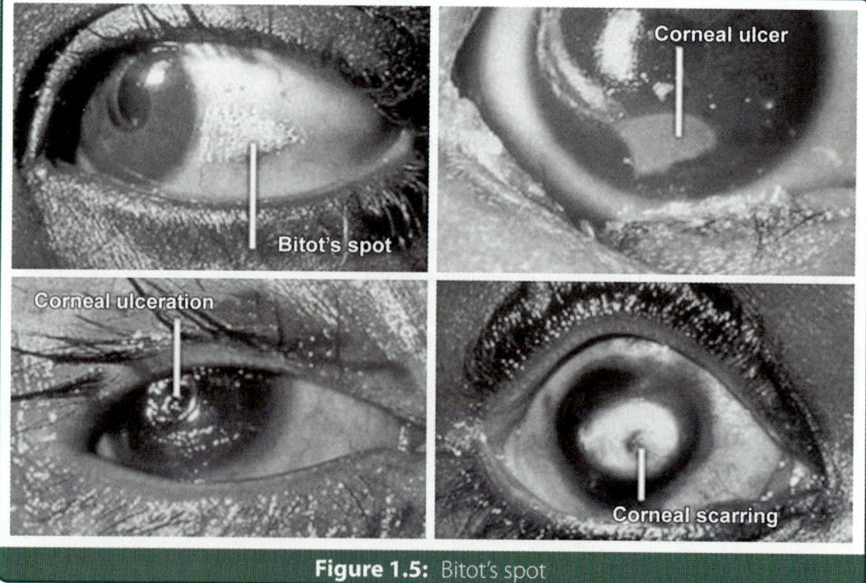

Figure 1.5: Bitot's spot

11. Why is there hypothermia?
    1. Edematous tissue—do not maintains heat preservation
    2. Skin changes
    3. Ulcers

    "common in kwashiorkor"
12. Gopalan's theory of adaptation and dysadaptation:

    Kwashiorkor and marasmus does not depend on qualitative or quantitative deficit of protein and calories. It is the response of (adaptation) the child to stress of undernutrition.

Principles of Gopalan's Theory

Flow Chart 1.1: Gopalan's Theory

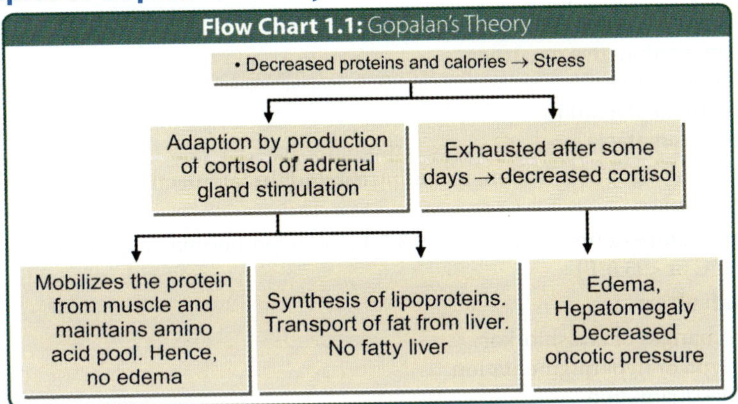

SEVERE ACUTE MALNUTRITION (SAM) (FIG. 1.6)

Weight for height/length <–3 z score of median of WHO child growth standards or bipedal edema.

If weight-for-height or weight-for-length cannot be measured, use the clinical signs for visible severe wasting.

History

- History examination
- Recent intake of food and fluids
- Usual diet (before the current illness)
- Breastfeeding
- Duration and frequency of diarrhea and vomiting
- Type of diarrhea (watery/bloody)
- Loss of appetite
- Family circumstances (to understand the child's social background)
- Chronic cough
- Contact with tuberculosis
- Recent contact with measles

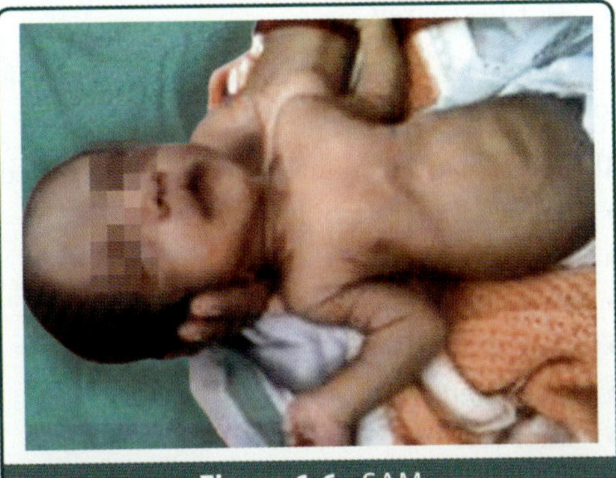

Figure 1.6: SAM

- Known or suspected HIV infection
- Immunizations

Examination

- Anthropometry—weight, height/length, mid-arm circumference
- Edema
- Pulse, respiratory rate
- Signs of dehydration
- Shock (cold hands, slow capillary refill, weak and rapid pulse)
- Severe palmar pallor
- Eye signs of vitamin A deficiency:
  - Dry conjunctiva or cornea
  - Bitot's spots
  - Corneal ulceration
  - Keratomalacia
- Localizing signs of infection, including ear and throat infections, skin infection or pneumonia
- Fever (temperature ≥37.5°C or ≥99.5°F) or hypothermia (axillary temperature <35.0°C or <95.0°F)·
- Mouth ulcers
- Skin changes of kwashiorkor:
  - Hypo or hyperpigmentation
  - Desquamation
  - Ulceration (spreading over limbs, thighs, genitalia, groin and behind the ears)
  - Exudative lesions (resembling severe burns) often with secondary infection (including candida)

Laboratory Tests

- Hemoglobin or packed cell volume in children with severe palmar pallor
- Blood sugar
- Serum electrolytes (sodium, potassium)
- Screening for infections:
  - Total and differential leukocyte count, blood culture (If possible)
  - Urine routine examination
  - Urine culture
  - Chest X-ray

There are 10 essential steps in two phases: An initial stabilization phase and a longer rehabilitation phase.

The focus of initial management is to prevent death while stabilizing the child

- Stabilization rehabilitation
- Hypoglycemia
- Hypothermia
- Dehydration
- Electrolytes
- Infection
- Micronutrients: No iron with iron

- Initiate feeding
- Catch-up growth
- Sensory stimulation
- Prepare for follow-up

World health organization guidelines in the management of SAM (severe acute malnutrition).

Treatment Guidelines

	Stabilization		*Rehabilitation*
	Days 1–2	*Days 3–7*	*Weeks 2–6*
1. Hypoglycemia	→		
2. Hypothermia	→		
3. Dehydration	→		
4. Electrolytes	→	→	→
5. Infection	→	→	
6. Micronutrients	No iron →	→	With iron →
7. Initiate feeding	→	→	
8. Catch-up growth			→
9. Sensory stimulation	→	→	→
10. Prepare for follow-up			→

Use of Antibiotics in SAM

Status	*Antibiotics*
All admitted cases	• Inj ampicillin 50 mg/kg/dose 6 hourly and Inj gentamicin 7.5 mg/kg once a day for 7 days • Add Inj cloxacillin 50 mg/kg/dose 6 hourly if staphylococcal infection is suspected • Revise therapy based on sensitivity report
For septic shock or worsening/ no improvement in initial hours	• IV Cefotaxime 50 mg/kg/dose 6 hourly or Inj cerftriaxone 50 mg/kg/dose 12 hourly plus Inj amikacin 15 mg/kg/once a day
Meningitis	• IV cefotaxime 50 mg/kg/dose 6 hourly or Inj cerftriaxone 50 mg/kg/dose 12 hourly plus Inj amikacin 15 mg/kg/once a day
Dysentery	• Inj ceftriaxone 100 mg/kg once a day for 5 days

Feeding Volume in SAM

Recommended schedule with gradual increase in feed volume is as follows

Days	*Freq*	*Vol/kg/feed*	*Vol/kg/day*
1–2	2 hourly	11 mL	130 mL
3–5	2 hourly	16 mL	130 mL
6 onwards	4 hourly	22 mL	130 mL

Starter Formula in SAM

Diets contents (per 100 mL)	*Starter formula*	*Starter formula (Cereal based) Ex: 1*	*Starter formula (Cereal based) Ex: 2*
Fresh cow's milk or equivalent (mL) (Approximate measure of one cup)	30 (1/3)	30 (1/3)	25 (1/4)
Sugar (g) (Approximate measure of one level teaspoon)	9 (1 + 1/2)	6 (1)	3 (1/2)
Cereal flour: Powdered puffed rice (g) (Approximate measure of one level teaspoon)	- -	2.5 (3/4)	6 (2)
Vegetable oil (g) (Approximate measure of one level teaspoon)	2 (1/2)	2.5 (1/2+)	3 (3/4)
Water: Make up to (mL)	100	100	100
Energy (kcal)	75	75	75
Protein (g)	0.9	1.1	1.2
Lactose (g)	1.2	1.2	1.0

Catch-up Formula in SAM

Diets contents (per 100 mL)	*Catch-up formula*	*Catch-up formula (cereal based) Ex: 1*
Fresh milk or equivalent (mL) (Approximate measure of one katori)	95 (3/4+)	75 (1/2)
Sugar (g) (Approximate measure of one level teaspoon)	5 (1)	2.5 (1/2-)
Cereal flour: puffed rice (g) (Approximate measure of one level teaspoon)	- -	7 (2)
Vegetable oil (g) (Approximate measure of one level teaspoon)	2 (1/2)	2 (1/2)
Water to make (mL)	100	100
Energy (kcal)	101	100
Protein (g)	2.9	2.9
Lactose (g)	3.8	3

Criteria for Discharge in SAM

	Criteria
Child	• Weight for height reached—ISD of median of WHO standards • Eating adequate amount of nutritious food that mother can prepare at home • Consistent weight gain • All vitamin and mineral deficiencies have been treated

Contd...

Contd...

	Criteria
	• All infections and other conditions have been treated or are being treated like anemia, diarrhea, malaria, tuberculosis • Full immunization program started
Mother or caretaker	• Able to take care of the child • Able to prepare appropriate foods and feed the child • Has been trained to give structured play therapy and sensory stimulation • Knows how to give home treatment for common problems and recognized danger signs warranting immediate medical assistance

Criteria for Early Discharge in SAM

	Criteria
Child	• Has a good apetite, eating at least 120–130 kcal/kg/day and receiving adequate micronutrients • Has lost edema • Consistent weight gain (at least 5 g/kg/day for 3 consecutive days) • Completed antibiotic treatment • Completed immunization appropriated for age
Mother or caretaker	• Trained on appropriate feeding • Has financial resources to feed the child • Motivated to follow the advise given

Forming the Diet Chart

Calorie Requirement

Immediately after birth: 150 kcal/kg (∴ At birth = 500 kcal)

Increase by 100 kcal/2 months up to 1 year

- 0 months = 500 kcal
- 2 months = 600 kcal
- 4 months = 700 kcal
- 6 months = 800 kcal
- 8 months = 900 kcal
- 10 months = 1000 kcal
- 12 months = 1100 kcal
- 1 year = 1100 kcals

  (Add by 100 kcal/year up to 5 years)
  - 1 year = 1100 kcal
  - 2 years = 1200 kcal
  - 3 years = 1300 kcal
  - 4 years = 1400 kcal
  - 5 years = 1500 kcal

5th year = 1500 kcal

6th year to 10th year: Male = 60–70 kcal/kg; Female= 50–60 kcal/kg

11/12 year: = 50–60 kcal/kg (male); 40–50 kcal/kg (females)

Holiday Sugar Formula

- <10 kg: 100 calories/kg
- 10–20 kg: Add 50 calories/kg to the previous
- >20 kg: Add 20 calories/kg to the above

Protein Requirement

- Normal: 2 g/kg BW
- PEM infant: 4 g/kg BW
  (or) 2 g/kg BW of expected weight

Cereals

Foof stuffs/preparation	Amount	Protein (g)	Calories (kcal)
Cooked rice	1 cup (100 g)	2	100
Wheat chapati	1	2	50
Pooris	2	2	50
Idly	1	2	50
White bread	1 slice	2	50
Dosai	1	2	50
Upma (rava/wheat)	1 cup	6	250
Barley (raw)	1 tsp	0.5	1.1
Ragi	6 tsp	2	100

1 cup–100 mL/100 g
1 tsp–5 mL/5 g
1 table spoon–3 tsp–15 mL/15 g
1 tumbler–2 cups–200 mL
1ounce (oz)–30 mL

Pulses

Food stuff	Amount	Protein	Calories
Cooked dal	1 tsp	1/2 (0.5)	15
Soya bean	100 gms	43	430
Bengal/green gram	1 tsp	1	18

Leafy Vegetables

Roots/Tubers

Araikeerai	100 g	2.8	44
Drum stick leaves	100 g	6.7	92
Beet root	100 g	1.7	48
Potato	100 g	1.6	97
Carrot	100 g	0.9	48
Radish	100 g	0.7	17

Milk/Milk Product

Food	Amount	Protein	Calories
Human milk	100 mL	1.1	65
Milk powder	1 tsp	2	18
Cow's milk	(100 mL)	1.3–3.5	60
Butter milk	10 Z (30 mL)	0.25	5
Curd	10 Z	1	20

Fruits and Other Vegetables

Food	Amount	Protein	Calories
Apple	100 g	0.2	60
Banana	100 g	0.6	50
Grapes	100 g	0.5	70
Guava	100 g	0.9	50
Lemon	100 g	0.7	35
Orange	100 g	0.7	60
Orange juice	100 g	0.2	10
Papaya	100 g	0.6	32
Brinjal	100 g	1.4	24
Cluster beans	100 g	3.2	60
Cucumber	100 g	0.4	10
Lady's finger	100 g	1.9	75
Johnston	100 g	1.4	21

Miscellaneous

Food	Amount	Protein	Calories
Ghee (cows)	1 tsp	0	45
Butter (salt)	100 g	0	730
Coconut	100 g	4.5	444
Cashewnut	100 g	21	600
Groundnut	100 g	26	570
Grand nut	100 g	9	200
Fish (shark)	100 g	22	0
Prawn	100 g	19	0
Fish (in general)	100 g	0	60
Beef	100 g	23	115
Pork	100 g	19	114
Goat	100 g	22	118
Egg (hen)	1 (50 g)	6–7	70–80
Biscuits	1	½	25

Contd...

Contd...

Food	Amount	Protein	Calories
Cane sugar	1 tsp	0	20
Brown sugar	1 tsp	0	15
Coconut water	100 mL	1.4	24
RISAM	1 cup	0	20
Coffee	1 cup	1.4	60
Ice cream	1 heaping	2	200
Oil	5 mL (1 tsp)	2	45

For Easy Remembering

Protein content:

- Cereals - 6.5–7 g%
- Rice - 6.4 g%
- Wheat - 12 g%
- 6 g of protein
  - 1 egg
  - 1 tumbler milk
  - 3 idlies
  - 3 chapati
  - 3 dosa
  - 3 bread slice
  - 12 tsp cooked dal
  - 1OZ meat/fish
  - 3 cups cooked rice
  - 50 groundnuts

Vegetables (100 g)	1 gram protein	50 kcal
Fruits (100 g)	½ gram protein	100 kcal
Meat 30 g = 1 egg		

How to write the Diet chart in exams?

Write 3 charts as shown below:

1. Before admission
2. At present in hospital
3. Recommended diet

Before Admission

Time	Food item and amount	Protein (G)	Calories
7 am 7.01–8.00 am	Milk 150 mL sugar 2 idlies/ghee 1 tsp		
1.00 pm			
4.00 pm			
8.00 pm 10.00 pm			
Total			

Balanced Diet: It is one which consists of all items of food like cereals, pulses, greens, etc. in optimum proportion for that age and sex with reserve for stressful period.

1. Energy derived from cereals not more than 75%
2. Ratio of cereal protein to pulse protein to be kept between 1:1
3. Minimum leafy 2 other vegetables not to exceed 150 g/day in adult
4. Minimum milk:100 mL/day
5. Energy from refined sugar: Kept around 5%
   Calories from fats/sugar not to exceed 20%
6. Level of food items suggested should be consumed by average child

When and why to introduce supplements/additional feeds (weaning)

After 4 months/beginning of 6th month

1. Pancreatic amylase appears
2. Baby starts drooling saliva that is ready to digest starch
3. Taste buds that are present from birth are connected to cortex
4. Chewing movements appear indicating neuromuscular coordination
5. Breast milk maximum level (600–700 mL) at 3 months:
   Thereafter no increase but there is a decrease gradually.
   So to satisfy the growth of baby, wean at 6th month.
6. Body store of Iron and vitamin A are exhausted by 6th month
7. Period of negativism after 6 months develops
   Therefore, food items that he will be taking in future should be given by small amounts after 6 months of age.

Weaning Foods

1. Weaning foods prepared with milk:
   a. Rice and milk payasam
   b. Green gram and milk payasam
   c. Carrot and milk as carrot kheer
   d. Dry banana powder and milk
2. Weaning foods without milk: Khichedi, idiappam and idli
3. Family diet modified and given to infants
   a. Rice and dal
   b. Pongal and Upma

Contraindications for Breastfeeding

1. Primary lactase insufficiency in infant (absolute CI)
2. Galactosemia in infant (absolute CI)
3. Active TB in mother
4. Serious ill health
5. Postpartum psychosis in mother
6. Mother on following drugs
   – Anticoagulants
   – Narcotics
   – Antineoplastic
   – Radioactive drugs

CASE 2 Abdomen

- Hepatosplenomegaly
- Hepatomegaly
- Splenomegaly
- Ascites

HEPATOSPLENOMEGALY

Main Causes

Infective

- Bacterial
  - Disseminated tuberculosis, SABE
  - Typhoid
  - Brucellosis
- Viral
  - Hepatitis (A, B, C, D, E)
  - Infectious mononucleosis
- Protozoal
  - Malaria
  - Kala azar
- Fungal
  - Histoplasmosis
- Miscellaneous
  - Syphilis
- Spirochete: Leptospirosis.

Congestive

- Congestive cardiac failure
- Right heart failure
- Portal hypertension
- Hepatic (or) portal vein thrombosis
- Hemolytic facies (Fig. 2.1).

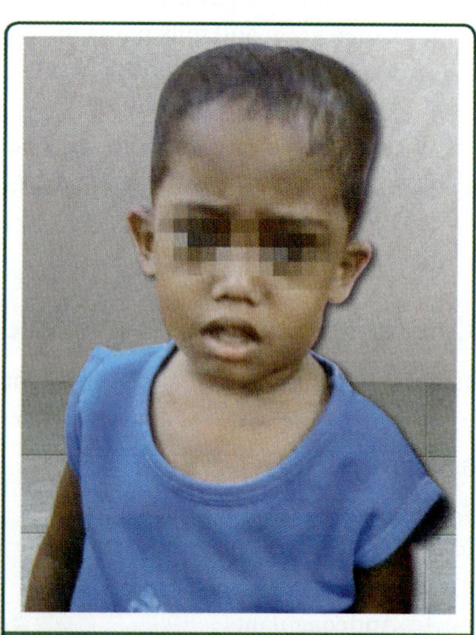

Figure 2.1: Hemolytic facies

Hematological

(Mostly splenomegaly)

- Hereditary spherocytosis
- Thalassemia
- Myeloproliferative disorders
- Sickle cell crisis

Infiltrative

- Leukemias

- Lymphoma
  - Hodgkin's
  - Non-Hodgkin's
- Liver
  - Fatty infiltration and secondary malignancies
- Primary malignancy (hepatomegaly).

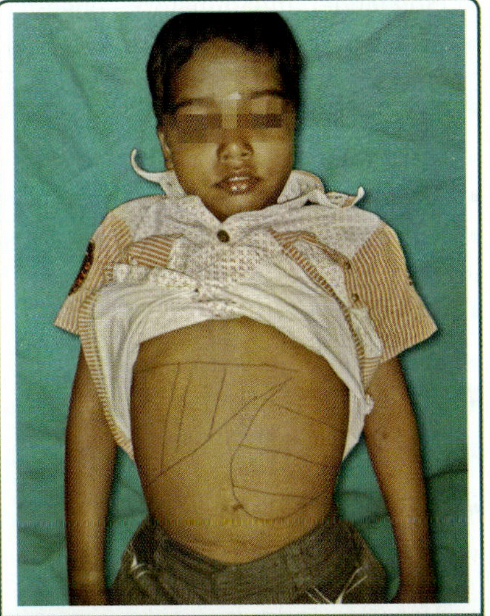

Figure 2.2: Glycogen storage disease (GSD)

Storage Disorder

- Glycogen storage diseases (Fig. 2.2)
- Niemann-Pick disease
- Gaucher's disease

Inflammatory and Collagen Vascular Disorder

- SLE and Rheumatoid arthritis

Miscellaneous

- Hepatomegaly:
  - Indian childhood cirrhosis portal hypertension
  - Gallstones
  - Kwashiorkor
  - Drugs—CCL_4, arsenic, chlorpromazine
  - Sarcoidosis
  - Amyloidosis
- Splenomegaly
  - Tropical massive splenomegaly (malaria)
  - Sarcoidosis
  - Amyloidosis
  - Iron deficiency
  - Thyrotoxicosis.

Practical Approach

Is liver really enlarged?

- Normally, it is felt upto 3 cm in infancy and childhood
- Apparent hepatomegaly (visceroptosis)
  1. Pneumothorax
  2. Bronchiolitis
  3. Emphysema
  4. Rickets
- Diagnosed by finding the upper border of liver (liver span).

Size

- Liver span: Height of liver in mid-clavicular line
- By percussion, the borders are made out.

Consistency

- Firm to hard: Chronic liver disease (CLD)

- Soft tender: Inflammatory/congested liver
- Isolated mass in normal liver: Tumor/cyst.

Age of Child

- Early Infancy—Neonatal cholestatis syndrome
- Preschool—ICC (Indian childhood cirrhosis)
- Older children and adolescent—Wilson's disease

Clues in the History

- Acute onset: Infective etiology
- Chronic (3–6 months)
  - Chronic active hepatitis
  - Cirrhosis
- Family H/O
  - Wilson's disease
  - Thalassemia
- Hepatotoxic drugs
  - Anti-TB, antiepileptic
  - Anticancer
- H/O needle pricks and transfusions—HBV/HCV

Clues in the Examination

- **Jaundice**: Viral hepatitis, active cirrhosis
- **Fever**:
  - Acute: Typhoid, malaria, leptospirosis
  - Chronic: Chronic active hepatitis, tuberculosis
- **Anemia**: Leukemia, hemolytic anemia, portal hypertension
- **Lymph adenopathy**: Disseminated TB, lymphoreticular malignancy
- **Neurological manifestations**: Wilson's disease, tyrosinemia.

Causes

Massive liver	*Massive spleen*	*Tender liver*
• Glycogen storage disorders	• Hypersplenism—Kala azar	• Viral hepatitis
• Congenital hepatic filariasis	• Extra hepatic PHT	• Congestive cardiac failure
• Tumor, cyst, abscess	• Chronic malaria	• Abscess
• Chronic extrahepatic cholestasis	• Hemolytic anemia	• Malignancy
	• Gaucher's disease	
	• Myelofibrosis	
	• Tropical splenomegaly—Malaria	
	• Chronic myelogenous leukemia (CML) (Juvenile)	

History Taking and Examination of a Abdomen Case

A 10-year-old......coming from......is brought to the hospital by the mother whose reliability is good.

- C/o
  - Fever past 15 days
  - Yellowish discoloration of urine 10 days
  - Abdomen distension (ascites)
  - Hematemesis
  - Melena
  - Abdominal pain.

History of Present Illness

1. Fever:
   - For past 15 days
   - Acute/chronic
   - High/low grade
   - Continuous/intermittent
   - Associated with chills/rigor
   - H/O Headache
2. Jaundice:
   - Past 10 days
   - Yellowish discoloration of eyes and mucous membrane
   - H/O High colored urine: Throughout - pathological
   - Early morning only—normal people (due to concentrated urine).

History in Liver Disorders

A. Appetite—liver disorders
   Abdominal pain (enzyme secretions ↓)

B. Bitot's spots : decreased bile and decreased absorption of fat-soluble vitamins
   Bowel symptoms (vomiting, diarrhea, constipation)

C. Cachexia/coma/convulsion (encephalopathy)

D. Distension of abdomen (hepatomegaly, peritonitis, ascites)

E. Ecchymosis (bleeding manifestations, decreased vitamin K, decreased II, VII, IV, X clotting factors

F. Fetor hepaticus (methyl mercaptan not metabolized and excreted)

G. Growth retardation/GI bleeding

H. Hair loss—(decreased, secretion of arginine, tyrosine essential amino acids), hematemesis

I. Itching; infections/NCS/obstructive bile pathology

J. Jaundice

K. Keratomalacia (dryness); kidney failure

L. Lassitude (decreased glycogen due to poor, absorption/conversion)

M.
   1. Melena
   2. Malnutrition
   3. Malabsorption
   4. Marasmus

N. Night blindness, neurological signs (flapping tremor)

O. Edema (hypoalbuminemia), Neonatal cholestatic syndrome (NCS)
P. Pruritus, pale stools—(H/O passing worms in stools)

Types of Fever

Continuous fever	*Remittent fever*	*Intermittent fever*
Does not fluctuate > 1 °C in 24 hours but never touches the normal	Daily fluctuation > 2 °C, never touches the baseline	Present only for several hours a day
For example: UTI, lobar pneumonia, typhoid, viral fever	For example: Enteric, bronchopneumonia	For example: Malaria, UTI, leptospirosis

Tertian fever—Appear on alternate days; *P vivax*
Quartan fever—2 days intervening between the attacks, *P malaria*
Quotidian fever—Intermittent fever that occurs daily
Pel-Ebstein fever—Hodgkin's disease
Saddleback fever—Dengue

Other Histories

- H/O vomiting
  - Content
  - Frequency
  - Color
  - Odor
  - Blood staining
- H/O Oliguria
  - Dysuria
  - Hematuria
  - Polyuria
  - Anuria

  } Hepatorenal syndrome
- H/O Cardiac problem
  - Dyspnea
  - Palpitation
  - Chest pain

  } Constrictive pericarditis: Ascites; Cardiac cirrhosis: Jaundice
- H/O Fever, rash arthritis: Collagen vascular disorders
- H/O Convulsions: Galactosemia
- H/O Blood transfusions
- H/O Drug intake
- H/O Fever > 6 months + bleeding manifestation: Leukemias/malignancy
- H/O Prolonged fever with double rise of temperature everyday: Kala azar

Past History

- Similar episodes
- TB/jaundice
- Exanthematous fevers
- Previous surgeries
- Previous hospitalization

Antenatal H/O:

Natal H/O: Neonatal jaundice, umbilical sepsis, catheterization, blood transfusion

Postnatal H/O:

Developmental H/O:

Diet H/O:

Immunization H/O: Fever—as for other

Family H/O: Importance of sibling, H/O—Reye's syndrome, Indian childhood cirrhosis, Wilson's disease

Contact H/O: Drugs—ATT

Negative H/O to be Elicited for Fever

- H/O Cough/nasal discharge – Recurrent respiratory infection
- H/O Ear discharge – CSOM
- H/O Sore throat – tonsillitis, pharyngitis
- H/O GI problems (vomiting, loose stools) – GI enteritis and peritonitis
- H/O Pyuria, hematuria, frequency, lower abdomen pain – UTI
- H/O Headache, projectile vomiting, neck stiffness – Meningitis
- H/O Rash, arthritis – Collagen vascular disorder
- H/O Bleeding manifestations + bone pain – Leukemias
- H/O periodicity – Malaria, kala azar
- H/O Body pain (Myalgia) – Leptospirosis
- H/O Joint pain + fever – Rheumatic fever

General Examination (Fig. 2.3)

- Conscious
- Cooperative
- Comfortable
- Anemic
- Jaundice
- Clubbing
- Cyanosis
- Pedal edema
- Significant lymph adenopathy
- Bony tenderness
- Dental caries
- BCG scar
- Signs of vitamin deficiency of A, D, E, K.

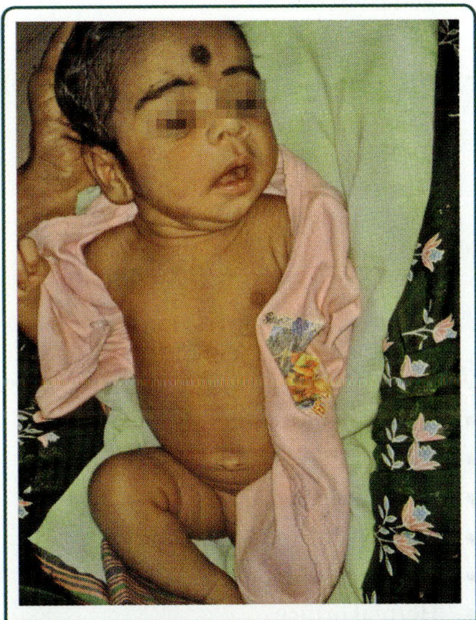

Figure 2.3 Neonatal cholestasis

Vital Signs

- Pulse
- BP
- Temperature
- RR.

Anthropometry

- Height
- Weight
- Head circumference

- Mid-arm circumference
- Chest circumference.

Head to Foot Examination

Signs of Liver Cell Failure

- Sparse hair
- Jaundice (Icteric)
- Vitamin A deficiency (Bitot's spot)
- Parotid enlargement
- Spider nevi
- Gynecomastia
- Anemia
- Fetor hepaticus
- Palmar erythema
- Dupuytren's contracture
- Leukonychia
- Pruritus
- Flapping tremor
- Caput medusae
- Abdomen distension
- Free fluid
- Pedal edema.

What are the things you see in hand?

1. Dupuytren's contracture
2. Palmar erythema
3. Flapping tremor
4. White nails
5. Anemia

Abdominal Examination

Inspection

- Shape of abdomen
- Skin, umbilicus, scar
- Dilated veins
- VGP/ visible pulsation
- Movement with respiration
- Hernial orifice
- External genitalia
- Flank full/not.

Palpation

- Warmth
- Soft, hard
- Tenderness
- Any mass

- Any organomegaly
- Fluid thrill
- If veins are see—note the direction of flow
- Renal angle tenderness
- Liver span (lower border).

Grading of Splenomegaly (Fig. 2.4 and 2.5)

- Mild—less than 3 cm
- Moderate—3–7 cm
- Severe—>7 cm.

Percussion

- Liver dullness (upper border)
- Traube's space
- Shifting dullness
- Tidal percussion.

Auscultation

- Bowel sounds
- Splenic rub
- Hepatic rub
- Venous hum
- Arterial bruit.

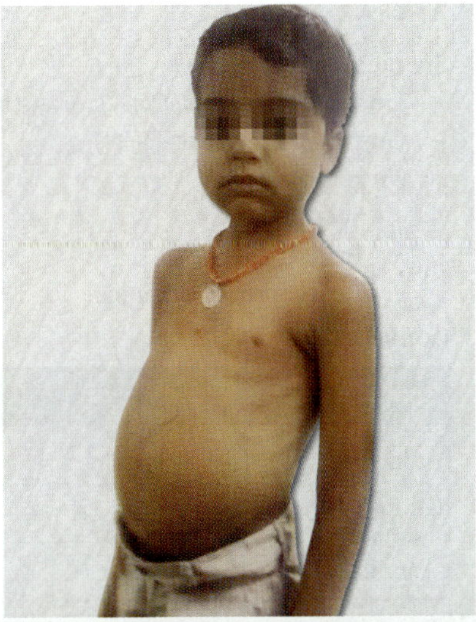

Figure 2.4 Massive spleen

Traube's Space Boundaries

- Superior—Left lung and diaphragm
- Inferior—Left subcostal margin
- Right—Left lobe of liver
- Left—Spleen

Obliterated in

- Full stomach
- Splenomegaly

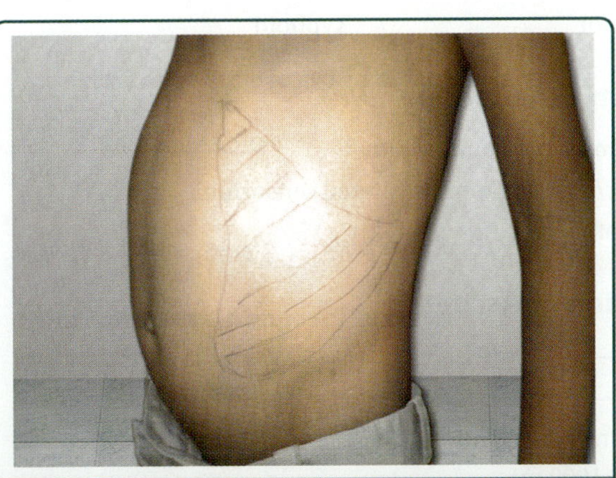

Figure 2.5 Extra hepatic portal vein obstruction

Physical Examination of Liver

1. **Size**:
   – Mild/moderate/severe
2. **Edge**:
   – Sharp
   – Thick
   – Rounded
   – Even/uneven
3. **Surface**:
   – Smooth: Hepatitis, CCF, storage disorders
   – Granular: Cirrhosis (ICC)
   – Uneven
     - Secondary
     - Primary
     - Postnecrotic cirrhosis
4. **Consistency:**

Soft	*Firm*	*Hard*
Fatty liver	Cirrhosis	• Congestive hepatic fibrosis
Kwashiorkor	Tuberculosis	• Postnecrotic macronodular cirrhosis
Anemia	Wilson's	• Malignancy
Septicemia	Galactosemia	
Push down liver	Tyrosinemia	
	Chronic liver disease	

5. **Tender liver:**

Liver abscess
CCF
Acute hepatitis
Primary tumor
Hydatid cyst
Post-invasive procedures
Percutaneous cholangiopancreatography
Typhoid

Other System Examination

- CVS: Heart murmur/venous hum
- CNS: tremor/flapping tremor/altered sensorium
- RS: Pleural effusion

Demonstration of Ascites

- Ultrasound—50–100 mL
- Puddle sign—150 mL
- Shifting dullness—500 mL
- Fluid thrill—1000 mL

Liver Span

Age	cm
Infants	5–6.5 cm
1–5 years	6–7 cm
5–10 years	7–9 cm
10–15 years	8–10 cm

Discussion

1. H/O Fever and splenomegaly
   - Soft spleen - Enteric fever
   - Firm spleen - Malaria
2. H/O Low grade fever and evening rise of temperature with splenomegaly and malnourishment with or without hepatomegaly
   - Disseminated TB
3. H/O Low grade fever and splenomegaly
   - Leukemia
   - Lymphomas (will also C/O Anemia, bone pain, bleeding tendencies)
   - With hepatomegaly/fever/rash : SLE/RA
4. Isolated splenomegaly
   - Chronic malaria
   - CML
   - Hairy cell leukemia
   - Extrahepatic portal hypertension
   - Cirrhosis and PHT (will have signs of liver failure)
   - Iron deficiency anemia
5. Hepatomegaly with anemia
   - Leukemia (ALL is common)
   - Chronic malaria
   - Hemolytic anemias
   - H/O Recent transfusion
   - Hemolytic facies (thalassemia)
6. Hepatomegaly with lymphadenopathy
   - Lymphomas
   - Disseminated TB
   - Infectious mononucleosis
   - Sarcoidosis
7. Isolated hepatomegaly
   - Acute viral infection
   - Hepatitis
   - Hepatic abscess
   - Cyst hydatid
   - AV malformation
   - Hepatomas and secondaries
   - CCF
   - Glycogen storage disease
   - Septicemia
   - Leptospirosis

8. Fever with abdominal pain:
   1. Viral hepatitis: If jaundice appears, fever disappears
   2. UTI: Due to cystitis
   3. Typhoid: Typhoid cholecystitis, gastritis
   4. Worm infestations: Colic pain.

Rare Causes

1. Henoch-Schönlein purpura, recurrent abdominal pain
2. Infantile polyposis
3. Abdominal type of epilepsy (without fever)
4. TB abdomen
   - Infants–serous ascitis
   - Older–ileocecal obstruction
5. Non-specific lymphadenitis
6. Rheumatic fever (very rare)

Nodes are Significant

- Axillary and cervical if size > 1 cm
- Inguinal if size > 2 cm
- Matted nodes

Epitrochlear nodes are seen in infectious mononucleosis and syphilis

HEPATOMEGALY

- C/O: Fever (high grade)
- Vomiting

Fever with rigor:

1. Malaria
2. Pneumococcal pneumonia
3. Upper UTI
4. Filariasis
5. Liver abscess
6. Cholangitis
7. Septicemia.

Fever with vomiting:

1. H/O Headache
   - Blurring of vision
   - Altered sensorium
   - Convulsion
   - Neck rigidity
   - **Diagnosis: Meningitis.**
2. Sudden onset of loss of consciousness
   - Refractory convulsions
   - **Diagnosis: Encephalitis.**
3. Drug induced: Chloroquine
4. Anorexia
5. Typhoid

Tender Hepatomegaly

1. CCF
2. Viral hepatitis
3. Liver abscess
4. Constrictive pericarditis
5. Pericardial effusion
6. Budd-Chiari syndrome
7. Veno-occlusive disease
8. Hepatoma

Hepatosplenomegaly Causes

1. **With fever:**
   - Malignancies
   - Hematological—AML, ALL (most common), CML
   - Infections
   - Collagen vascular disorders
   - Cholangitis
   - Chronic active hepatitis
2. **With jaundice:**
   - Chronic active hepatitis—hepatitis A, B, C, D, E
   - Cirrhosis with portal hypertension
   - Infectious mononucleosis
   - Leptospirosis (due to hemolysis and obstruction)
   - Septicemia
3. **With anemia:**
   - Chronic malaria (hemolysis)
   - Cirrhosis with portal hypertension (bleeding varices)
   - Malignancy (bone marrow depression)
   - Fumigant sepsis (disseminated intravascular coagulation)
4. **With lymphadenopathy:**
   - Lymphomas
   - Leukemias
   - IMN
   - TB
   - Sarcoidosis
5. **With bleeding manifests:**
   - Cirrhosis and PHT
   - Purpura
   - Intrauterine infections
   - Hepatitis
   - Hematological malignancy
6. **Neurological manifestations:**
   - Wilson's
   - Glycogen storage disorders
   - Encephalopathy
   - CNS tuberculosis

How can you say it is a chronic liver disease?

- Clinically: Long duration and firm liver
- Albumin level : Low, i.e. <2.5 = Duration >30 days
- Prothrombin time prolonged
- A:G ratio reversed

DIFFERENTIAL DIAGNOSIS

Typhoid Fever

Points in favor: (C/O Frontal headache (more specific)

1. Spleen (3–4 times enlarged)
2. Fever and vomiting
3. Peripheral healing/central coating of tongue
4. Alternating bowel habits
5. Tender hepatomegaly
6. Rashes (rose spots).

Investigations

1. Culture:
   - Blood culture = Ox bile broth medium (not to be done if on antibiotics like ciprofloxacin)
   - Urine culture
   - Stool culture
2. Blood widal (after 7 days)
3. Blood:
   - TC—Leukopenia (not specific) (<5,000: Pediatric)
   - Initial 1st week—Lcukocytosis (>14,000: Pediatric)
   - DC—Lymphocytosis (late stages)
   - Platelet count decreased
   - Anemia
   - Increased basophils
   - Toxic granules in polymorphonuclear leukocytes
4. PCR—most specific: Positive in cases inadequately treated and vaccinated.

Blood Widal (Tube Agglutination Test)

Serological test to detect antibodies to *Salmonella* infection in the serum of suspected case

- **Specimen**
  - Blood collected at end of I week (after 7 days)
  - 2 mL of serum to be separated for test
- **Reagents**
  - Antigen H and O of *S typhi*
  - Antigen 'A' of para 'A'
  - Antigen 'H' of para 'B'
  - Saline as diluents

- **Glass wares**
  - Dreyer's tube: Conical bottomed for 'H'
  - Felix tube: Round bottomed for 'O'
  - Slit lamp

Doubling dilution of serum is used:
For example, in 25/1, in 50/1, in 100.......etc.

- **B—Blood positive in 1st week**
- **A—Antibody serology widal in 2nd week**
- **S—Stool positive in 3rd week**
- **U—Urine positive in 4th week**

Carriers—more dangerous

- Somatic 'O' specific for typhoid
- 'H' antigen—Non-specific (also raised in *Yersinia*)

Start treatment when widal + at 1/160; 1/320 dilutions.

Complications of Typhoid Fever

- I week: Meningism (typhoid encephalopathy)
  - Toxic
  - Anorexia
  - High fever
  - Transient neck stiffness
- II week: Typhoid bronchitis (not responds to reaction)
- III week: Intestinal perforation, peritonitis and hemorrhage
- IV week:
  - Carrier state
  - Osteomyelitis
  - Septic arthritis
  - Myocarditis
  - CSOM (3rd week–4th week).

Stages of Typhoid

1. **Prodromal stage: 1 week:** Period of invasion
   - C/O: Malaise, headache
   - Abdomen pain, constipation, diarrhea
2. **Fastigial stage: II and III week:** Continuous fever
   - Child quite ill
   - Pea soup stools
   - Coma
   - Distended abdomen
   - Spleen+
   - Rales+
   - Apathy, stupor, delirium

3 **Defervescence stage:**
   - Condition improves
   - Normal temperature: 7–10 days
   - Child more alert, symptoms disappear
   - Relapses more common at this stage

Complication

1. GIT:
   - Poor orodental hygiene
   - Hemorrhage
   - Perforation
   - Peritonitis
   - Sepsis
   - Overt hepatitis, liver abscess, fatty liver
   - Cholecystitis
   - Pancreatitis
2. Lungs:
   - Pneumonia
   - Bronchitis
   - Pulmonary infarct
3. CVS:
   - Toxic myocarditis, arrhythmias, cardiogenic shock
   - Endocarditis
   - Thrombosis/phlebitis
4. CNS:
   - Increased ICT: Cerebral venous thrombosis
   - Acute cerebellar ataxia
   - Aphasia, deafness, psychosis
   - Transverse myelitis
   - Optic neuritis
   - Meningism
   - Apathy
   - Typhoid encephalopathy (loss of abdomen reflex—earliest sign)
   - Sequelae (rare)
5. Renal:
   - Pyelonephritis
   - Nephrotic syndrome
   - Cystitis and pyelitis
6. Skin: Furuncles and bed sores
7. Ortho: Septic arthritis
   - Osteomyelitis
8. Miscellaneous: Otitis media
   - Parotitis
   - Suppurative lymphadenitis
   - Orchitis
   - Alopecia
   - Uveitis
   - Hemorrhagic typhoid
9. Relapse: In 6 weeks

Diagnosis of Typhoid Perforation

1. Abdomen distension
2. Toxic
3. Rigidity
4. Absent bowel sounds
5. Guarding/tenderness
6. X-ray: Air under diaphragm.

Management

- General:
  - Good diet
  - Bed rest
- Chloramphenicol—50 mg/kg/day (TDS/QID) (14 days)
- Adverse effects:
  - Aplastic anemia
  - Agranulocytosis
  - Grey baby syndrome.

MDR Typhoid

Criteria: Plasmid-mediated resistance and the organism does not responds to

1. Chloramphenicol
2. Ampicillin
3. Cotrimoxazole
4. Amoxicillin

Treatment : Ciprofloxacin- 10 mg/kg BW IV for 10–14 days
Latest treatment regimen:

- Ceftriaxone IV.

Treatment of Encephalitis

- Admit ICU
- Electrolyte Balance
- 7.5 mL/kg mannitol
- Dexamethasone: 3 mg/kg 6th hourly, 8 doses
- Cephalosporins: 3rd generation
- Anticonvulsants.

Indication of Steroids

- Minimal steroids:
  - (When patient is still toxic and not responds)
  - 0.1–0.2 mg /kg body weight
  - H_2 blockers.

Treatment of Carrier State

- Amoxicillin (or) ampicillin-specific (4–6 weeks) because they accumulate in bile and enters GIT.

Other Drugs

- Ceftriaxone IV
- Ciprofloxacin IV
- Chloramphenicol: It is not effective, since it does not reach urinary tract
- Treatment of relapse/quinolone resistant: Azithromycin.

Tuberculosis

- Prevalence—2%
- C/O
  - Loss of appetite
  - Failure to thrive
  - Anorexia
  - Cervical adenopathy
  - Persistent cough.

Post-primary Complex

In poor community persons, primary complex goes for

1. Reactivation
2. Extension to surrounding regions
   - Pleurisy
   - Dissemination
   - Consolidation.

Treatment

- I line:

Rifampicin(R)	- 10–15 mg/kg single dose oral
Isoniazid(H)	- 5–10 mg/kg oral
Streptomycin(S)	- 20–30 mg/kg (maximum 1 g) IM
Ethambutol(E)	- 25 mg/kg oral
Pyrazinamide (Z)	- 20–35 mg/kg oral

- II line:

Ethionamide	- 15 mg/kg oral
Ciprofloxacin	- 10 mg/kg oral
Amikacin	- 7.5 mg/kg/day (divided) IV/IM

Latest Diagnostic Tools

- Sputum smear for microscopy
- Chest X-ray
- Sputum culture and DST for diagnosing drug resistant TB
- Newer rapid diagnostic tools for MDR/XDR TB.

Sputum Microscopy

- Simple, specific, reliable, feasible, correlates with infectivity sputum specimens
  1. Gastric juice
  2. Induced sputum
  3. Bronchoalveolar lavage.

Chest X-ray

- More sensitive
- Less specific
- Higher inter and intrareader variation
- No shadow is characteristic of TB
- 10% false negative
- 40% false positive .

Mantoux Test

- Used to diagnose infection by tuberculin
- 1, 2 and 5 tuberculin unit (TU)
- Efforts should be made to use 1TU and in no case strength higher than 5 TU should be used
- The current cutoff of 10 mm cannot be justified for strength higher than 5 TU, degree of necrosis and ulceration may not necessarily differentiate infected from diseased.

Interferon Gamma Release Assay

Measures production of interferon gamma by peripheral mononuclear cells.

Quantiferon gold and T-spot test

- Expensive, do not differentiate TB infection from disease
- Exact utility in high burden countries still not clear.

Culture Methods

- Solid medium—LJ medium
- Liquid medium:
  - Bactec [radiometric]
  - MGIT [non-radiometric]
- MGIT
  - Mycobacterial growth indicator tube system
  - Detects growth as early as 4 days after inoculation
  - DST will be available in 21–28 days.

Polymerase Chain Reaction (PCR) Test

- Detects presence of resistance genes
- Do not differentiate live or dead bacilli
- No decisions can be made only with PCR
- Currently, not recommended in clinical practice.

Serodiagnostic Tests

- No specific antigen
- Neither confirms nor differentiate infection
- Both antigen and antibody TB enzyme-linked immunosorbent assay (ELISA) tests are poorly sensitive and specific
- Not recommended for diagnosis of tuberculosis.

Histopathological Examination

- For extrapulmonary forms
- FNAC helps to confirm TB when clinical presentation not typical
- Biopsy do not have place in routine clinical practice
- Caseating necrosis, granuloma, epithelioid cells, giant cells

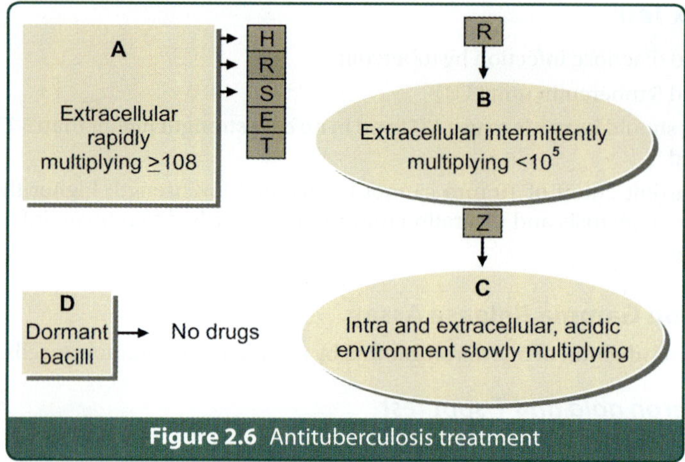

Figure 2.6 Antituberculosis treatment

Other Tests

- Complete blood count
  - Neutrophilic?
  - Lymphocytosis?
  - ESR-non-specific.

Treatment

- Scientific basis
- Antituberculosis treatment (ATT) and sub-bacillary population (Fig. 2.6).

Intermittent SCC-LAG Period

"When a colony of *Mycobacterium tuberculosis* (MTB) is exposed to anti-TB drugs, TB stops multiplying for a variable period 2–40 days [lag phase] before new growth occurs".

Revised national tuberculosis control program (RNTCP) utilizes this lag phase and ATT given intermittently as DOTS.

Categorization of Patients

- New case—category I
  [Formerly category I and category III]
- Previously treated case
  [Formerly category II]
- New case:—A TB patient who has never had treatment for TB or has taken ATT for less than one month
  [Formerly category I and category III].

New Case Treatment

- $2\,H_3R_3E_3Z_3/4H_3R_3$
- Intensive phase: 8 weeks [24 doses]
- Continuation phase: 18 weeks [54 doses]
- If sputum positive at the end of 2 months, IP is continued for another month, i.e. 12 more doses

New Cases Treatment Continue

- For TBM cases injection SM is used in place of ETM in intensive phase
- So 2 $H_3R_3S_3Z_3$ instead of 2 $H_3R_3E_3Z_3$
- For TBM and spinal TB 7 months of CP
- So total duration is 9 months instead of 6
- Steroids in TB definite—TB meningitis, TB pericarditis

May be used in:

- Endobronchial TB
- Mediastinal compression
- Immune reactivation syndrome, pleurisy with respiratory distress.

Previously Treated Case

- Relapse
- Failure
- Default
- Previous category II.

Treatment Regimen Previously Treated Cases

- Intensive phase 2 $S_3H_3R_3E_3Z_3$/1 $H_3R_3E_3Z_3$
- Continuation phase 5 $H_3R_3E_3$
- Total duration 8 months

If sputum is positive at the end of 3 months, IP extended for another 1 month 12 doses.

Relapse > Failure and Default

Patientwise Drug Boxes

- Red color—New
- Blue color—Previously treated
- Intensive phase 1 blister = 1 day
- Continuation phase 1 blister = 1 week
- No other DOTS program in the world has patient wise box (PWB) for children with TB.

Pediatric PWB with Dosages

Drugs	*Early bactericidal*	*Sterilizing activity*	*Prevention of emergence of drug resistance*
Isoniazid	++++	++	++++
Rifampicin	+++	++++	+++
Streptomycin	+++	-	++
Pyrazinamide	++	+++	+
Ethambutol	+	-	++

PWB for New Cases According to Weight Band

Drug Resistant TB

- Multidrug resistant TB [MDR-TB]
- Resistance to at least isoniazid and rifampicin
- Extensively drug resistant TB [XDR-TB]
- MDR-TB plus resistance to a fluoroquinolone and at least one of three injectables [amikacin, capreomycin and kanamycin]
- Standardized treatment regimen for MDR-TB
  RNTCP Category IV Regimen
  Supervised Daily single Dose regimen

Latent Tuberculosis Infection: Chemoprophylaxis

- < 6 Years
- Positive Mantoux
- Intrafamilial contact
- INH 5 mg/kg for 6 months
- Available tablet 100 mg of INH.

Newborn to a Mother with TB

- Do not withheld BCG vaccine
- Continue breastfeeding
- Prophylactic INH for 6 months for newborn
- Separation of infant from mother not necessary.

The Difference Category III is Phased out

- Merged with category I
- Ethambutol can be used in all age groups.

Older Regime

Treatment schedule for pediatric tuberculosis:
DOTS is the recommended strategy for treatment of TB, and all pediatric TB patients must be registered under RNTCP.

Category of treatment	*Type of patients*	*Intensive phase*	*Continuation phase*
Category I	• New smear positive pulmonary TB • Seriously ill sputum smear negative pulmonary TB • Seriously ill extrapulmonary TB*	2 $H_3R_3Z_3E_3$	4 H_3R_3
Category II	• Sputum smear positive relapse • Sputum smear positive treatment failure	2 S_3 $H_3R_3Z_3E_3$/ 1 $H_3R_3Z_3E_3$	5$H_3R_3E_3$
Category III	• Sputum smear negative • Extrapulmonary TB , Not seriously ill**	2 $H_3R_3Z_3$	4 H_3R_3

***: Seriously ill extrapulmonary TB** indicates disseminated TB/Miliary TB, TB pericarditis, TB peritonitis and intestinal TB, bilateral extensive pleurisy, spinal TB with or without neurological complications, genitourinary TB, bone and joint TB
****: Not seriously ill** indicates lymphnodes and unilateral pleural effusion.

Indications for Steroids

A. Pleural/peritoneal involvement
B. Segmental
C. Ocular
D. Lymph nodes with sinus
E. Miliary/disseminated
F. TB meningitis/tuberculoma
G. Genitourinary
Prednisolone 1 mg/kg
Single dose 4–6 weeks and tapper.

Genitourinary

Same dose: 8–12 weeks and taper.

Leptospirosis

- C/O Severe myalgia of calf muscles
- Conjunctival suffusion
- Spleen+
- Liver+, jaundice and oliguria
- Causative organism: *Leptospira interrogans*
- Source: Infected rat urine
- Mode of entry: Direct (eroded skin) or indirect (contaminated urine).

Investigation

- Early diagnosis: IgM ELISA (2nd day)
- Microslide agglutination (Positive after 7–10 days)
- Urine culture
- Phase contrast microscope.

Treatment

- Injection benzylpenicillin 6–8 lac unit/kg BW for 7 days
- If allergic to penicillin doxycycline 8–10 mg/kg single dose.

Malaria

- C/O Intermittent fever (3/2nd days)
- Chills/rigor
- Firm spleen (splenohepatomegaly).

Investigation

- Peripheral smear for MP
- PCR.

Treatment

Uncomplicated

- Chloroquine—10 mg base/kg stat, 5 mg/kg at 6, 24, 48 hours
- Primaquine—0.25 mg/kg/day - for *P vivax* and ovale along chloroquine for 14 days.

Chloraquine Resistant Falciparum

- Artesunate—4 mg/kg for 10 days
- Sulfadoxine—20 mg/kg + Pyrimethamine - 1 mg/kg single dose
- ACT regimen—Artesunate combination therapy.

Both resistant

- Mefloquine—15 mg/kg 1st dose: then 10 mg/kg in (8–24) hours
- Mefloquine resistance—Halofantrine 8–15 mg/kg BW single dose for 5 days
- Artemisinin—(3.2 mg/kg/day BW for 6 days)

Chemoprophylaxis

- *P falciparum*—Proguanil and pyrimethamine
- *P vivax*—Pyrimethamine

Dengue Fever

- Interval of 48 hours in between the fevers—saddleback fever or break-bone fever.
- I phase—similar to other viral fever
- II phase—Bone pain
  - Rashes
  - Altered sensorium
  - Dehydration

Investigation

- Rapid antigen estimation
- No culture medium
- Antibody titer
- R_X: ORS/fruit juice
  - Paracetamol (when >39°C)
  - Metabolic/electrolyte balance
  - O_2 administration
  - Non-hepatotoxic sedatives—chloralhydrate (12.5–50 mg/kg)

Consolidation of Investigations for an Abdomen Case

Preliminary

1. Complete blood count:
   - To diagnose the type of anemia
   - To diagnose the leukemia
   - To diagnose the infection
2. Reticulocyte count—Increased in hemolytic anemia
   - Normal—<1%
3. Tuberculosis screening:
   - Mantoux test
   - RGI: Ryle's tube aspiration and gastric juice for acid-fast bacteria (AFB) staining
   - Chest X-ray
   - USG abdomen
4. Liver function test
   - SGOT: Increased in acute viral hepatitis
   - SGPT: Liver specific

- Alkaline phosphatase: Increased in obstructive jaundice
- Prothrombin time: Increased in liver cell failure
- Total proteins: Decreased in chronic liver disease
- Viral markers: HBsAg, anti-HAV IgM, HBeAg, HBV DNA copies

5. Blood grouping for urgent transfusion
6. Blood glucose for glycogen storage disorder
7. VDRL
8. TORCH screening
9. Blood culture for sepsis cases

Specific Investigations

1. Leptospirosis
   - Dark ground microscopy
   - MSAT/MAT
   - Urine /blood culture
2. Tuberculosis
   - PCR
   - BACTEC
   - IgM for TB cell wall
   - Adenosine deaminase test
3. HIDA scan
   - For liver: Extrahepatic biliary atresia
4. USG
   - Liver
   - Portal vein flow
   - Dilated ducts
5. Duodenal aspirate for bile
   - Chronic active biliary disease
6. Liver biopsy
   - Chronic hepatitis

Accelerated BCG Test

Normal BCG: Left arm at the level of insertion of Deltoid BCG vaccine is given.

Inference

Pneumonic-PANUS

Weeks

- 4—Papule
- 5—nodule
- 6—ulcerates/heals
- 8—scar
- Accelerated BCG: Given in right arm
- Based on hypersensitivity to tuberculin protein
- Result: Formation of papule, nodule and pustule in 24–72 hours.

Hypersensitivity BCG: <24 hours (or) < 1 day
Classical accelerated: 24–72 hours (or) 2–3 days
Delayed accelerated: >72 hours – 7 days (or) 3–7 days

CASE 3 Cerebral Palsy

CASE FORMAT

Complaints

- Delayed milestones
- Delayed head control.

Present Illness (Ask for Developmental Milestones)

- Social smile
- Head control
- Rolling over
- Reaching to object
- Sitting
- Crawling
- Standing
- Walking

1. Bladder/bowel control
2. Language
3. Fine motor and pick up small things
4. High-pitched cry
5. Playing

- H/O: Floppy on lifting [atonic cerebral palsy (CP)]
- H/O: Stiffness of limbs (e.g. crossing of legs)
  - On holding in the hip
  - Scissoring gait of spastic cerebral palsy (CP), difficulty in applying diapers
- H/O: Paucity of movements of limb/weakness of limbs
- H/O: Convulsions
- H/O: Involuntary movements (basal ganglia lesions)
- H/O: Regression of attained milestones (neurodegenerative disorders)
- H/O: Suggestive of increased ICT (seizures, irritability, vomiting and headache)
- H/O: Higher function
  - Recognizing mother
  - Orientation
  - Interest in surrounding
  - Sleep patterns
  - Behavioral pattern.

History Suggestive of Cranial Nerves Dysfunctions

- Recognizing parents/able to reach object: 2nd nerve (optic nerve)
- Squint/abnormal eye movements: 3rd, 4th and 6th nerve
- Facial asymmetry, difficulty in mastication, drooling of saliva: 7th nerve (facial nerve)

- Responds to call and sounds: 8th nerve (vestibulocochlear)
- Nasal regurgitation/feeding difficulties/weak cry: 9th, 10th and 12th nerve—H/O aspiration
- Deviation of tongue to any side: 12th nerve (hypoglossal nerve)
- H/O Sensory involvement: Response to pain/temperature
- H/O Motor involvement: Limb involvement
- H/O Suggestive meningitis: Fever; lethargy, convulsion, seizures, neck rigidity.

Antenatal History

- Child is born to a 25-year-old mother/2nd baby regular antenatal checkups
- Booked and immunized case; iron and folic acid tablet given
- H/O Antepartum hemorrhage (asphyxia)
- H/O PIH (IUGR)
- H/O Exanthematous illness
- H/O Drug intake
  - Propranolol: IUGR
  - Quinine: CNS anomalies
- H/O Jaundice; fits (PIH)
- H/O Irradiation: Microcephaly, mental retardation
- H/O Previous BOH
- H/O Maternal diabetics: Birth asphyxia, hypoglycemia, hyperbilirubinemia
- H/O Teratogenic drugs

Natal History

- Preterm/term/post-term
- Domiciliary/hospital: Normal full-term delivery
- Prolonged 2nd stage
- Birth weight
- Cried immediately or late
- History of keeping child in neonatal ICU
- Breastfeeding: After how many hours
- If late, why?
- Mode of delivery
  - Vaginal
  - Cesarean: Indication—fetal distress/CPD
  - Liquor clear or not

Postnatal History

- H/O Asphyxia
- H/O Convulsions
- H/O Jaundice
- H/O Any drug intake
- H/O Immunization
- H/O Flabbiness
- H/O Feeding difficulties

DEVELOPMENTAL HISTORY

- Typical H/O: Mother noticed stiffness of limbs, particularly lower limbs. No other abnormal movements.

Gross Motor

- 3 months: Neck holding
- 5 months: Sitting with support
- 8 months: Sitting without support
- 9 months: Standing with support
- 10 months: Walking with support
- 11 months: (Crawling at 8th month) (creeping-10th month)
- 12 months: Standing without support
- 13 months: Walking without support
- 18 months: Running
- 24 months: Walking upstairs (Both feet on same step) (at 3 years with alternate steps)
- 36 months: Riding tricycle.

Fine Motor

- 4 months: Grasps a ring when placed in hand
- 5 months: Bidextrous grasp by intentional reaching
- 7 months: Palmar grasp
- 9 months: Pincer grasp (Holds small objects between index and thumb).

Language

- 1 month: Turns head to sounds
- 3 months: Cooing
- 6 months: Monosyllables (ma, ba)
- 9 months: Bi syllables (mama, baba)
- 12 months: Two words with meaning
- 18 months: Ten words with meaning
- 24 months: Simple sentence
- 36 months: Tells story (5 lines).

Personal/Social

- 2 months: Social smile
- 3 months: Recognizes her mother
- 6 months: Smiles at mirror image
- 9 months: Waves bye-bye
- 12 months: Plays a simple ball game
- 36 months: Knows gender.

Bladder/Bowel Control

Pneumonic for Milestones

LOX- STD
235-456

L: Line—2nd year
O: Circle—3rd year
X: Cross/plus—5th year
S: Square—4th year
T: Triangle—5th year
D: Diamond—6th year

DIETARY HISTORY

- Breastfeeding how long? Times/day
- Any difficulty
- H/O Aspiration while feeding
- H/O Weaning
- Calculate calorie/protein intake/requirement

Immunization History

- Family and social history
- H/O Similar illness in family = Degenerative disorder of brain

GENERAL EXAMINATION

- Conscious/awake/looking around/interested in surroundings
- Neurocutaneous markers
- Posture/attitude
- Smiling or inappropriate laughter.

Posture

- Lying down
- Legs crossing over one another
- Extended legs
- Upper limbs flexed: Shows choreoathetoid movement

Appearance

- Not looking at us
- Not aware of surroundings
- Any other voluntary/involuntary movement

Cutaneous markers: Café au lait spots, Ash leaf macules, adenoma sebaceum, etc.
Congenital anomalies: Pallor/icterus/cyanosis/clubbing/pedal edema/lymph node

Head

- Microcephaly (less than 3 SD)
- Shape of skull
- Anterior and posterior fontanelles/sutures.

Limbs

- Short limbs
- Cortical thumb.

Eyes

- Cataract/squint/hypertelorism nystagmus.

Mouth

- Drooling saliva.

Gait

- Contractures
- Scissoring
- Flat foot.

VITAL SIGNS

Respiratory rate

- Newborn: 40–60/minute
  - 1 year: 30–40/minute
  - 5 years: 20/minute
  - 10 years: 18/minute

Heart rate

- Newborn: 140/minute
  - 1 year: 110/minute
  - 3 years: 100/minute
  - 8 Years: 90/minute
  - 10 years: 80/minute

Blood pressure

- Newborn: 65/45 mm Hg
  - 1 year: 75/50 mm Hg
  - 3 years: 90/60 mm Hg
  - 8 years: 95/65 mm Hg
  - 10 years: 100/70 mm Hg

Temperature

- >5 years: Take oral temperatures
- <5 years: Groin/axilla/rectum
  - N: 36.5–37.5°C
- >41°C is hyperpyrexia
- Axilla/groin: 0.5°C less than oral
  - Rectal: 0.5°C higher than oral

EXAMINATION OF CENTRAL NERVOUS SYSTEM (FIG. 3.1)

Higher Functions

- Alert, awake, responds/not responds to stimuli
- Speech/handedness/memory/language/orientation to person, time, place
- Interested in surroundings.

Examination of Cranial Nerves

I (Olfactory nerve): Not tested

II (Optic nerve) Vision: Recognizable parents

- Fixing of objects
- Color vision
- Visual acuity
- Pupillary reflex
- Fundus examination

III/IV/VI (3—oculomotor/4—trochlear/6—abducens nerves)

- Follows the object
- Squint
- Doll's eye movement, extraocular movement

(Doll's eye movement: Moving head to one side eye ball moves to other side)

L/F: Ptosis

- Dilated pupils
- Diplopia
- Divergent squint

V N: (Trigeminal nerve)

- Sensation over face (not possible in children)
- Muscles of mastication

VII N: (Facial nerve)

- Deviation of angle of mouth
- Nasolabial furrow obliteration

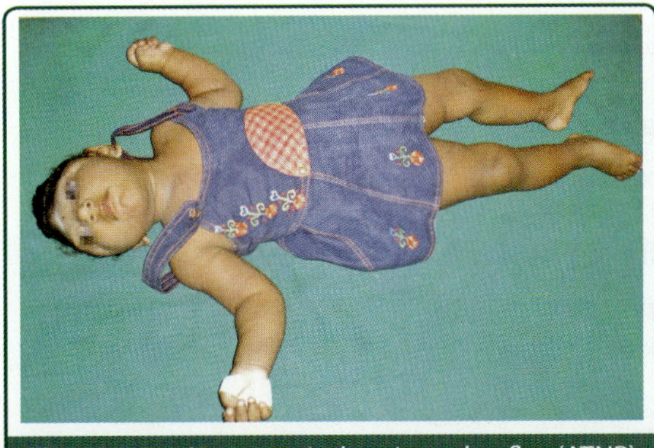

Figure 3.1: Asymmetrical tonic neck reflex (ATNR)

- Closing of eye
- Wrinkling of fore head
- Buccinator weakness
- Taste: Anterior 2/3 tongue

VIII N: (Vestibulocochlear nerve)

- Hearing

IX/X N: (9—glossopharyngeal, 10—vagus nerve)

- Gag reflex
- Uvula position

XI N: Turning of head to one side

XII N: (Hypoglossal nerve) Movements of tongue/wasting of tongue/fasciculations, fibrillations.

Spino-Motor System

- Nutrition
- Bulk
  - Compare both sides for wasting/hypertrophy
  - Measure mid-arm/mid-thigh circumference
  - Palpate the muscle for flabbiness
- Tone: Check by passive movements
- Power: See the hand movement by giving some object

MRC grading of muscle weakness:

- Complete paralysis
- Visible flicker
- Move while eliminating gravity
- Move against gravity
- Move against resistance
- Normal

- Reflexes: Deep/superficial
- Autonomic system.

Autonomic System

- Bladder/bowel control.

Sensory/Cerebellar

- No need to examine.

Neonatal Reflexes (Refer Page No. 169)

- Moro: Disappears by 3 months
- Rooting/sucking
- Grasping
- Palmar grasp

- Asymmetric
- Glabellar tap
- Crossed extension
- Palmomental reflex

Gait

- Scissoring gait

Spine

- Normal

Grading of Reflexes

- Absent
- Present (normal ankle jerk)
- Brisk (normal knee jerk)
- Very brisk
- Clonus

Other Systems

- CVS: S_1S_2+, no murmur
- RS: NVBS
- Abdomen: P/A soft, no organomegaly

Points Favoring

- Exaggerated reflexes
- Increased tone
- Extensor plantar response after 1 year
- Persistence of primitive neonatal reflexes
- Delayed milestones/not attained milestones
- Small head size/regression of head circumference (Figs 3.2)
- Cortical thumb (Figs 3.3)

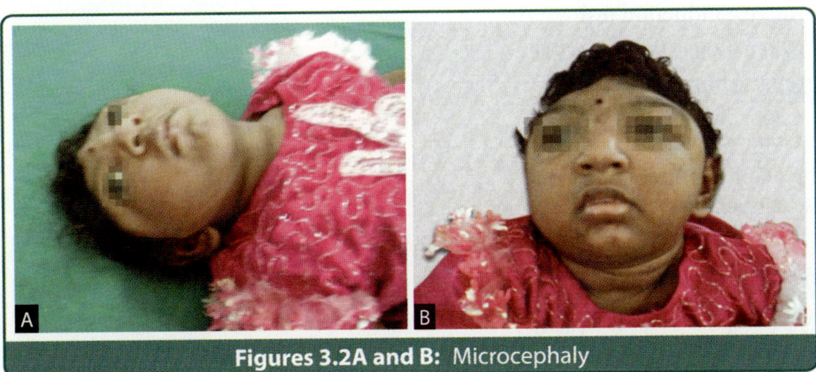

Figures 3.2A and B: Microcephaly

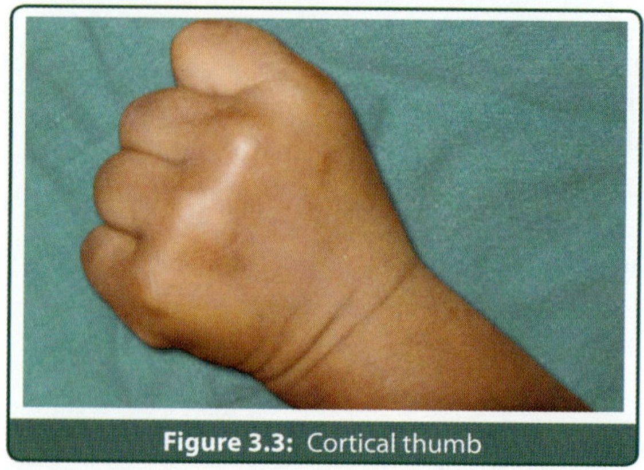

Figure 3.3: Cortical thumb

Diagnosis

Spastic cerebral palsy: Quadriplegia and mental retardation with microcephaly with protein energy malnutrition.

Investigations

- Screening for the TORCH
- Urine examination to find out the preventable cause of mental retardation:
  - Phenylketonuria
  - Galactosemia
  - Hypothyroidism (thyroid function study)

> Benedict's test: Galactosemia
> Ferric chloride test: Phenylketonuria
> Cyanate nitroprusside: Homocystinuria
> Cetrimide: Mucopolysaccharides

- Neurosonogram
  - Ultrasonogram through the anterior fontanelle
- CT Scan
- MRI
- EEG
- EMG
- Nerve conduction test
- Nerve biopsy (sural nerve)
- Muscle biopsy
- Assessment:
  - ENT: Hearing test
  - Ophthalmology: Vision
  - Psychiatry: IQ
  - Physiotherapy
- Thyroid function test
- Chromosomal analysis
- Vision/hearing/speech assessment.

Management

Team work containing the following specialists with pediatrician as head:

1. Surgeon/orthopedician
2. ENT surgeon
3. Ophthalmologist
4. Speech therapist
5. Neurologist
6. Psychiatrist
7. Psychologist
8. Educator
9. Social worker
10. Mother/father
11. Physiotherapist

Surgeon/orthopedician

- Tendo Achilles lengthening
- Synovectomy for adductor tendons (adductor spasm)
- Rhizotomy (cutting sympathetic fibers)
- Tendon transfer procedures.

ENT surgeon: Hearing appliances
Ophthalmologist: Correct squint
Optometrist: Correct astigmatism
Speech therapist: Training
Neurologist: Carbamazepine
Sodium valproate for seizures
Psychiatrist: Convince the parents/counseling
Educator: Play therapy
Social worker: Coordination
Physiotherapy: Galvanic current stimulation.

Grade I: Normal school: Copy the habits from others
Grade II: Special schools: Special school with play therapy
Grade III: Parental accompany to special schools
Grade IV: Institutional management
Training minimum basics: eat, toilet, etc.

CEREBRAL PALSY

It is a non-progressive neuromotor disorder with or without involving vision, speech, hearing due to lesion of developing brain.

Classification

I. **Physiological:**
   - Spastic (increased tone)
   - Athetoid (involuntary movements)
   - Atonic
   - Ataxic (incoordination)

- Rigid (extrapyramidal)
- Mixed
- Unclassified (not coming under above)
- Tremor present

II. Topographic:

- Monoplegia: One limb
- Diplegia: All 4 limbs/but lower 2 limbs more involved
- Triplegia: Any 3 limb
- Quadriplegia: All 4 limbs equally involved
- Hemiplegia: One side/more of upper limb
- Double hemiplegia: Both half of body involved more of upper limb
- Paraplegia: Only lower limb

III. Etiological:

- Prenatal
- Natal
- Postnatal

Prenatal	*Natal*	*Postnatal*
Infection (STARCH)	Anoxia (predominant)	Trauma
Metabolic	Difficult labor	Meningitis
Toxemia (PIH)	Precipitated labor	Infection
Infarction	Sedatives given to mother	
Genetic	Asphyxia	
Anoxia	Hypoxia	
Irradiation		

IV. Grading:

- No negligible loss of functions
- Mild to moderate loss
- Moderate to severe loss
- No purposeful activity

V. Clinical:

- Spastic hemiplegia
- Spastic diplegia
- Spastic quadriplegia
- Atonic
- Extrapyramidal
- Mixed.

Etiology

I. Prenatal

1st Trimester: TORCH infection

T: Toxoplasma

O: Others—Syphilis
H zoster
HIV-AIDS
TB
Varicella
Other exanthems

R: Rubella
C: CMV
H: HSV- II (Genital)

STARCH Complex:
S: Syphilis
T: Toxoplasma
A: AIDS
R: Rubella
C: CMV
H: HSV

II. Ingestion of drugs
   - Anticonvulsants
   - Alcohol
   - Antithyroid
   - Oral hypoglycemic
   - Reserpine
III. Radiation:

IInd Trimester

Placental insufficiency: IUGR

(PIH, Infarcts)

IIIrd Trimester: APH (placenta)
- Example
- Epileptic fits
- Premature placental separation.

For all trimester:
- Anemia
- Diabetes
- Hypertension

Natal

- Anoxia: Kinking or pinching of umbilical cord
- Asphyxia: Block of respiratory passage
- Analgesia: To the mother—affects the respiratory center of baby. Fetal asphyxia-damage to brain
- Difficult labor: CPD, strenuous application of forceps
- Breech presentation
- Sudden change in pressure: Example, precipitate labor and cesarean section
  - Results in sudden release in pressure, hence, there is insufficient time for the natural decompression with resultant emboli and rupture of blood vessels.
- Premature: More liable, since blood vessels are weak
  - Predispose to cerebral hemorrhage
  - Premature babies: USG
  - Hypoechoic
  - Periventricular areas

  Strong predictor of later development of motor dysfunction

- Birth weight:
  - Low birth weight (cerebral diplegia): <1000 gm—intracerebral hemorrhage and periventricular leukomalacia
  - Normal birth weight: Quadriparesis or hemiparesis

Postnatal

- Kernicterus (Athetoid CP)
- Trauma: Skull fracture
- Infection: Meningitis and encephalitis
- Vascular: Hemorrhagic—thrombosis and embolism

Ingram's Classification

I. Spastic: 74%
   a. Diplegic
   b. Hemiplegic
   c. Rigid or spastic

II. Ataxic: 13%
   a. Simple cerebellar
   b. Diplegic

III. Dyskinetic: 5.5%
   a. Choreoathetoid
   b. Trauma

IV. Minimal: 4.8%
   a. Clumsy child
   b. Behavioral disorder

V. Mixed: 2.6%

Other Types

1. **Dyskinetic CP:** (Extrapyramidal) athetoid CP
   Dyskinetic include: Athetosis, choreiform, tremors, rigidity
   MR present: Hearing defect seen
2. **Hypotonic CP:** Atonic CP
   - Hypotonia with poor head control and lag
   - Rare form, mostly head lag represent an evolving form of dyskinetic or spastic CP
   - DTR, Normal or brisk always; Babinski +
   - Severe mental retardation
   - DD cerebellar involvement: (hypotonic with DTR not exaggerated)
3. **Ataxic CP:**
   - Hypotonia and hyporeflexia
   - Ataxia and intention tremor by 2 years
   - Intellect: Normal (rare nystagmus)
   - Wide-based gait
   - Ataxic: May be associated with spasticity (ataxic diplegia)

Associated Features

1. **Mental retardation:** (50–75%)—Common in spastic quadriplegia (atonic CP)
2. **Seizures:** (25–33%)—Often in spastic hemi/quadriplegia. Least in dyskinetic CP

Table 3.1: Differences in features between the types of cerebral palsy

Features	*Spastic Hemiplegia*	*Spastic Diplegia*	*Spastic Quadriplegia*	*Athetoid*
CT scan	Cortical white matter degeneration with dilatation of lateral ventricles	Periventricular leukomalacia	Widespread cortical white matter degeneration with cystic cavity formation	Kernicterus (basal ganglia) Hypermyelination of basal ganglia
Moro reflex	Asymmetrical	Both lower limb component absent (partial moro)		
Tone	Increased	Increased		Atonic CP
Deep tendon reflex	Increased	Increased	Spasm of all four limbs	Despite hypotonia, DTR are normal or brisk
Clonus	+	+		
Plantar reflex	Extensor Babinski +			Babinski + as it is UMN lesion
Hand preference (Holding with right hand, if object is given)	Normal—3 years < 1 year They obtain it by 6 months			
Gait	Shortening of tenco Achilles Hence, unilateral tip toe walk Circumduction gait	Unable to turn over Bilateral tip toe walk	Autoregulation is lost	Shake and see the baby Floopy infant

Contd...

Contd...

Features	*Spastic Hemiplegia*	*Spastic Diplegia*	*Spastic Quadriplegia*	*Athetoid*
Mental retardation/seizures	25% have MR 1/3rd have seizures	No mental retardation/ convulsions	Severe MR/seizures/contractures common	No head control Drooling saliva Falls forward
Milestones	Delayed in motor and mental milestones	Mental milestones normal Delayed motor milestones	Vision/speech and hearing impaired	No MR Cortex and medulla—normal Relatively intelligent
		C/o inability to carry by mother Commando walk (crawl)	No growth of brain. Both milestones absent 6th nerve commonly involved—Longest intracranial nerve 8/10/11—drooling saliva/ regurgitation and dysphasia	Normal mental milestones Delayed motor milestones Neonatal jaundice with Hyperbilirubinemia

3. **Ears:** (15–20%)—Partial/complete loss of hearing usual in kernicterus.
   Brain damage due to rubella. (receptive auditory dysphasia)
4. **Speech:** Aphasia, dysarthria, dyslalia, common in dyskinetic CP
5. **Eyes:** (50–70%)—Strabismus paralysis of gaze, cataract, coloboma, retrolental fibroplasias, refractive error
6. **Behavior problems**: (30–50%)—Stubbornness, aggressiveness, lack of attention and hyperkinetic behavior
7. **Sensory deficit**: Astereogenesis, spatial disorientation
8. **Others**: Inadequate thermoregulation.

Investigations

- Urine examination:
  - For PKU- Ferric chloride
  - Benedicts test for galactosemia
- X-ray skull:
  - Microcephaly
  - Calcification: Patchy (Toxoplasma)
  - Periventricular (CMV)
  - Rail road (tram line): Sturge-Weber syndrome
- CT scan
- MRI
- EEG: To find seizure
  - General/focal: Spastic group
  - Myoclonic: Akinetic/dyskinetic
- Nerve conduction study/nerve biopsy
- Muscle biopsy/EMG
- Metabolic screening test
- Vision
- Hearing: High tone audiometry
- Speech
- Psychometric and sensory evaluation
- Chromatography of (plasma and urine): Exclude inborn errors of metabolism

Differential Diagnosis

1. Neurodegenerative disorders: Progressive, familial, consanguineous parents
   - C/O: Failure to thrive
   - Regression of attained milestones
   - Vomiting
   - Seizure
2. Hydrocephalus and subdural effusion: Head size large, AF bulges, separation of sutures
3. Brain tumors/SOL: Progressive; features of increased ICT
4. Muscle disorders: Myotonia congenita
   - Hypotonia, decreased reflexes
   - EMG, muscle biopsy, increased CPK level
5. Ataxia telangiectasia: Family H/O
6. Minimal brain dysfunction syndrome

Viva Questions

1. How will you suspect congenital intrauterine infections?

a. Newborn child with fever, rash, hepatosplenomegaly
b. Mental retardation, convulsions, lymphadenopathy

2. What is the use of Apgar score?

a. At 1 minute = For resuscitation
b. At 5–10 minutes = Predicted the neurological outcome

3. Posture:

a. Hypotonic: Pithed frog position
b. Hypertonic: Opisthotonus posture (or) extended limb

4. Neurocutaneous markers:

a. Sturge-Weber syndrome: Port-wine, nevi of face
   (Cortical atrophy)
b. Neurofibromatosis (optic glioma, meningitis and acoustic neuroma)
   Café au lait spots:
   Significance:
      1.5 mm size > 5 numbers (preadolescent)
      15 mm size and > 6 numbers (adolescent)
c. Tuberous sclerosis: Ash leaf macules; shagreen patches; adenoma sebaceum

CEREBRAL PALSY: LITTLE'S DISEASE

Definition

It is a static encephalopathy that may be defined as a non-progressive disorder of posture and movement often associated with epilepsy, and abnormalities of speech, vision and intellect/resulting from a defect or lesion of the developing brain.

- Full development of brain = 2 years
- First described by Little, an orthopedician

Incidence: 2/1000

Epidemiology/Etiology

- Primary causes:
  - Birth trauma
  - Asphyxia (10%)
  - Prematurity

Classification

- Already written

Spastic Hemiplegia

- Have decreased spontaneous movements
- Hand preference earlier
- Walking is delayed (18–24 months)
- Circumduction gait
  - Extremities show growth arrest

  - (Particularly hand and thumbnail)
  - Particularly, in lesion involving contralateral parietal lobe.
- Spasticity of the affected extremity is evidenced by equinovarus deformity
- Tiptoe walk: Is seen of increased tone
- Upper limb assumes: Dystonic posture when child runs
- 1/3rd: Seizure disorder (first year or two); 25%—mental retardation.

CNS finding:

- Ankle clonus +
- Babinski +
- DTR increased

} affected limb

CT scan:

- Atrophic cerebral hemisphere with dilated lateral ventricle contralateral to the side of affected extremities
- Intrauterine thromboembolic: Manifest as an area of focal cerebral infarct. Present with focal seizures at birth.

Spastic Diplegia

Bilateral spasticity of legs
First indication is noted when child begins to crawl.
Child uses arm as a normal manner but tends to drag the body behind as a military man; rather than using four limbs (Commando crawl).

On examination:

i. Severe adduction at thighs (unable to apply diaper)
ii. When child is suspended by axial 'Scissoring posture' of lower extremities
iii. 'Equinovarus' both foot; 'Tip toe walk' both foot
iv. Walking is delayed.

   CNS finding:
   - Deep tendon reflex increased
   - Babinski +
   - Ankle clonus

   } Bilateral

v. Lower limb wasting with good stretching of upper limb (Disuse atrophy).

Salient points:

- Seizure—minimal
- No mental retardation.

CT Scan

- Periventricular leukomalacia, particularly of fibers apparent to lower limbs.

Spastic Quadriplegia

- Most severe form
- Marked motor impairment of all extremities
- Marked high mental retardation
- Maximum with seizures

C/O: Aspiration pneumonia
Due to swallowing difficulty owing to 'supranuclear bulbar palsy: 9/10th nerve palsy.

On examination:

- Increased tone
- Spasticity
- Spontaneous movements
- DTR increased
- Bilateral plantar extensor
- Flexion contractures of knees elbows by late childhood.

Salient features:

- Development disabilities, speech and visual abnormalities
- Have evidence of athetosis (may be classified mixed CP).

CT Scan:

- Cystic cavity.

Autopsy:

- Central white is disrupted by areas of necrotic degeneration that may coalesce into cystic cavities.

Athetoid

- Relatively rare
- Due to aggressive management of hyperbilirubinemia and kernicterus; it is rare nowadays.

On examination:

- Hypotonic
- Poor head control
- Marked head lag.

C/O: Feeding difficulty

- Tongue thrust
- Drooling prominent.

Salient features:

- Athetoid movements may not become evident until 1 year age and tend to coincide with hypermyelination of basal ganglia.
  (Status marmoratus)
- Speech is typically affected (oropharyngeal muscles are involved)
  - Slurred
  - Impaired voice
  - Modulation
- UMN signs:
  - Seizures
  - Intellect normal.

Viva

When will you suspect CP? Or what are the early markers of CP?

Suspect CP, if the infant has any one of following:

1. **Seizures:**

   In the 1st week of life, not accounted for other causes and reappearing during infancy and during episodes of respiratory and other-infections/not attaining time appropriate milestones.

2. **Reflexes:**
   - Rooting/Sucking: Sluggish in the 1st week of life
   - Moro/grasp/tonic neck: Present beyond 3 months of life
   - Stepping reflex: Absent in first 2 months
3. **Movements:**
   - Poverty or asymmetry of movements during kicking and playing in a cradle
   - Poverty of finger movements while handling a toy
   - Hand preference
4. **Posture:**
   - Stiffness during passive movement
   - Scissoring of lower legs (de Lange's sign).
5. **Cortical thumb: '*Critchley's sign*'**
   - Uncontrollable/intolerable cry
   - Normal cortical thumb persists <1 month
   - If >1 month; think of CP
6. **Decreased head size.**

Why there are feeding difficulty in CP?

- **Spastic type:** Tight sphincter → Aspiration pneumonia
- **Athetoid/atonic type:** Difficult of swallow
- **Quadriplegia:** Bulbar palsy

How will you assess muscle tone as a marker of cerebral palsy?

Should be assessed in alert/awake baby

- Abnormal posture
- Palpate muscles see whether flabby/firm
- Range of movements and resistance
- Shaking the unsupported limb (passive movements)

How will you assess the range of movement?

- Adductor angle
- Popliteal angle
- Dorsiflexion of angle of foot
- Heel to ear movement
- Scarf sign
- Parachute response (absent in spastic CP)
- Landau reflex (absent in floppy CP)

Adductor Angle

Infant lies supine legs extended and head in midline, both hips are abducted maximally by holding the knees with index finger

- Angle between thighs measured
- Asymmetry between R/L noted.

Popliteal Angle

Supine infants, hips are flexed completely on the abdomen by holding at knees. The legs are then extended by gentle pressure with examiner's hand placed behind legs and

- Measure popliteal angle
- Both side resistance.

Dorsiflexion

- Passively dorsiflexed by gentle pressure over sole
- Measure angle between dorsum foot and front of leg.

Heel-Ear Maneuver

- With infant lying supine: Legs extended at knees are held together and lifted as possible towards the ear : Without lifting pelvis.
- Inference: Note increased resistance on one side.

Scarf Sign

Upper limb flexed elbow pulled as for possible across chest by holding at the hand and wrist

Age	*Adductor angle (degrees)*	*Popliteal angle (degrees)*	*Dorsiflexion (degrees)*	*Scarf Sign*
(Months)				
0–3	40–80	80–100	60–70	Elbow do not cross midline
4–6	70–110	90–120	60–70	Crosses midline
7–9	110–140	110–160	60–70	Crosses anterior axillary line
10–12	140–160	150–170	60–70	

History for Seizures

1. **Febrile convulsions**
   - H/O Fever and infection
   - H/O Mode of onset
   - Number of episodes
   - H/O Vaccination +
   - Family History
   - Any H/O Postictal deficit
   - Any H/O Pertussis vaccination
2. **Grand mal epilepsy**
   - H/O Aura
   - H/O Tonic phase
   - H/O Clonic phase
   - H/O Postictal phase (post epilepsy)
   - H/O Todd's Palsy (<24 hours)

   H/O aura:
   - Auditory
   - Visual
   - Tactile
   - Sensory
   - Motor
   - Autonomic

H/O Tonic phase: (30 sec)

- Rigidity in antigravity muscles
- H/O Unconsciousness
- H/O Eye rolled upwards/fixed
- H/O Frothing mouth
- H/O Bladder/bowel emptied
- H/O Shrill cry (laryngeal muscles +)

3. **Atonic-akinetic**

   Consciousness lost but returned immediately.

   Atonic: H/O Sudden loss of muscle tone in limb, trunk, neck .

   Akinetic: H/O Movement lost; but not tone

4. **Status epilepticus**

   (Seizure lasts beyond 30 minutes not regaining conscious in between)

   - H/O Loss of consciousness in between the attacks.

5. **Status convulsivus**

   Child becomes conscious in between attack

   H/O Neurological deficit after attacks (9% cases)

Classification of mental retardation:

- Mild: 51–70
- Moderate: 36–50
- Severe: 27–35
- Profound: 0–20

Borderline Intelligence: 71–90

- Educatile: Mild
- Trainable: Moderate
- Custodial: Severe and profound

Management of Cerebral Palsy

I. **Physiotherapy**:

Physio-occupational therapy

(After developmental assessment)

'Bobath technique'

To reduce spasticity

- Prevent abnormal posture
- Promote motor milestones
- Stimulation of sensory, cognitive, perceptional functions
- Training in activities of daily life
- Treat associated problems
- Prevent contractures and deformities
- Special education

II. **Treatment of spasticity**:

Drugs: (pneumonic-BAD-BD)

- Baclofen: Dose 1.25–2.5 mg BD orally
  Increase upto maximum: 20 mg/day
  Function—depresses both mono and polysynaptic reflexes
- Alcohol (dilute)
  At motor points of nerves
- Diazepam: Spasticity and athetosis
- Dantrolene sodium: Relaxation of skeletal muscles
- Botulinum toxin.

III. **Surgical:**
- Obturator neurectomy
- Adductor tenotomy
- Psoas transfer and release
- Posterior rhizotomy
- Lengthening of tendo Achilles.

IV. **Other treatments:**
- Behavioral disturbance: Transquilizers
- Seizures: Anticonvulsants
- Athetosis: Levodopa
- Dystonia: Carbamazepine (or) Trihexyphenidyl)
- Sialorrhea: Benztropine/atropine
- Release of tongue tie
- Parotid duct transplantation into maxillary sinus for drooling of saliva
- Splints for cortical thumb

V. Occupation rehabilitation

VI. Educational: Typewriters/special computer

VII. Speech Rx

VIII. Ophthalmologist

IX. Hearing aids

X. Counseling

XI. Follow up

CASE 4 Renal System

DIFFERENTIATION BETWEEN NEPHRITIS AND NEPHROTIC SYNDROME

Nephritist	*Nephrotic syndrome (Fig. 4.1)*
1. Incidence:	
School age (6–12 years)	Preschool (2–6 years)
2. H/O Infection	
H/O Sore throat	
H/O Skin infections	
3. **Clinical features:**	
Acute onset	Insidious onset
Mild to moderate edema	Massive
Hematuria +	-
Oliguria +	Oliguria +
Hypertension +	-
4. **Investigations:**	
Urine	
i. RBC's and RBC Casts	Hyaline casts
ii. Spot urine:	
$\left.\frac{\text{Protein}}{\text{Creatinine}}\right\} 0.3-3$	>3
iii. 24 hr urine	
1+	3+
2+	4+
iv. Albumin: Trace	50 mg/kg/day 40 mg/m^2/ h
Blood:	
1. Total serum protein: Normal	Decreased(<5g/ dL)
2. Serum albumin: Normal	(<2.5 g/dL)
3. A:G ratio: Normal	Reversal
4. Cholesterol: Normal	>220 mg/dL
5 Electrophoresis: Normal	Decreased albumin ; α_2-globulin
X-ray chest:	
• Cardiomegaly	Hydrothorax
• Congested lung fields	(Transudate)
USG Abdomen:	
Renal enlargement	Kidney not enlarged

Contd...

Contd...

Nephritist	*Nephrotic syndrome (Fig. 4.1)*
Treatment: • Salt restricted diet and rest • Penicillin: 10 days • Treat hypertension: Calcium-channel blockers • Diuretics	**Treatment:** • Rest/fluid/salt restricted diet • Diuretics • Steroids—prednisolone for 4–6 weeks • Cyclophosphamide (Immunosuppressants)
Complications: • Acute renal failure • Hypertension • Electrolyte disturbance (Increased K^+ and PO_4^- Decreased Ca^{2+}) • Acidosis • Seizures	**Complications:** • Infections (Spontaneous peritonitis) • Arterial/venous thrombosis • Ascites/pleural effusion

HISTORY TAKING

- Age : School going children (5–8 years—AGN)
- Young children (3–8 years—Nephrotic)
- Sex: More among boys
- Place
- Informant: Mother
- Reliability: Good

C/O

1. Puffiness and face
2. Oliguria
3. High-colored urine
4. Abdomen distention.

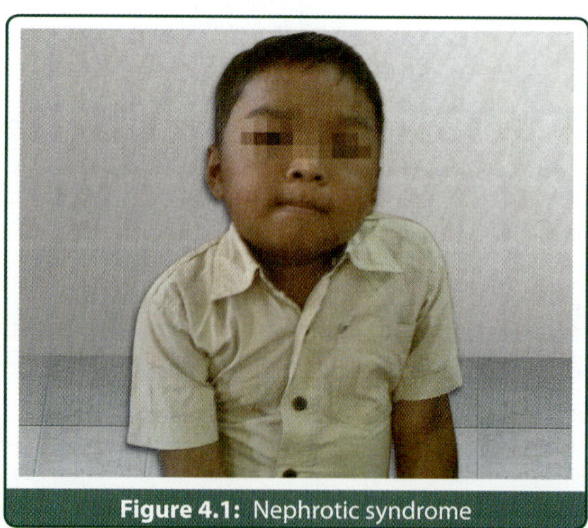

Figure 4.1: Nephrotic syndrome

DD: EDEMA

1. Renal causes:

   Edema starts in face: more in morning
   1. AGN
   2. Nephrotic syndrome
   3. Acute/chronic renal failure
   4. Urinary tract infection
2. Cardiac causes:

   Edema -***more in feet and sacrum (dependent***)
   1. CCF
   2. Pericarditis
   3. Pericardial effusion
3. Hepatic causes:
   1. Ascites
   2. Cirrhosis with PHT
4. Nutritional edema:
   - Kwashiorkor
   - Beriberi
5. Endocrine cause:
   - Cushing syndrome
   - Hypothyroidism
6. Collagen vascular disorders:
   - SLE
7. Superior mediastinal syndrome:
8. Angioneurotic edema:

   Ask H/O to rule out all causes:
   - H/O Pharyngitis, skin infection
   - H/O Oliguria
   - H/O Red/cola colored urine
   - H/O Breathlessness
   - H/O Chest pain, palpitation, orthopnea, paroxysmal nocturnal dyspnea (CCF)
   - H/O Abdomen pain, loss of appetite, jaundice -liver causes
   - H/O blurring vision, nausea, vomiting, convulsions (hypertension/hypertension encephalopathy)
   - H/O Recurrent RTI
   - H/O Dysuria,UTI
   - H/O Fever, rash, abdomen pain, arthritis (connective tissue disorders)
   - H/O Jaundice (hepatic encephalopathy)
   - H/O Ear discharge (secondary to streptococcal pharyngitis)
   - H/O Deafness (Alport's syndrome—deafness with hematuria).

PAST HISTORY

- H/O Similar illness before (nephrotic syndrome has 2–3 episodes before but rare in AGN)
- H/O Steroid therapy (nephrotic syndrome)
- H/O Skin infections—common in summer
- H/O Sore throat (post-streptococcal/glomerulonephritis)—common in winter
- H/O TB

- H/O Ear discharge
- H/O Exanthematous fever/measles—IgA nephropathy

- **Antenatal/natal/postnatal-history**:
- **Developmental history**: In PEM
- **Diet history**: To r/o PEM producing edema (kwashiorkor)
- **Family history**: Similar illness: among family members social economic states
- **H/o Siblings with infection**: Surrounding area of living and over crow cling
- **Immunization history**: BCG vaccine
- **Contact history**: Tuberculosis, sore throat.

GENERAL EXAMINATION

- Conscious
- Cooperative
- Nourishment
- General Appearance: Puffy face with periodical edema (Fig. 4.2)
- Anemia, other vitamin deficiency
- Jaundice, clubbing, cyanosis
- Lymph adenopathy (Jugulo-digastric node)
- Pedal edema
  - Minimal edema- AGN
  - Massive (anasarca)—nephrotic/PEM

Look for - **previous impetiginous scar**: Cause for acute glomerulonephritis.
Examine—throat, tonsil, ear, scalp.

Vital Signs

- Pulse
- BP (sometimes labile hypertension in AGN)
- Temperature
- Respiratory rate.

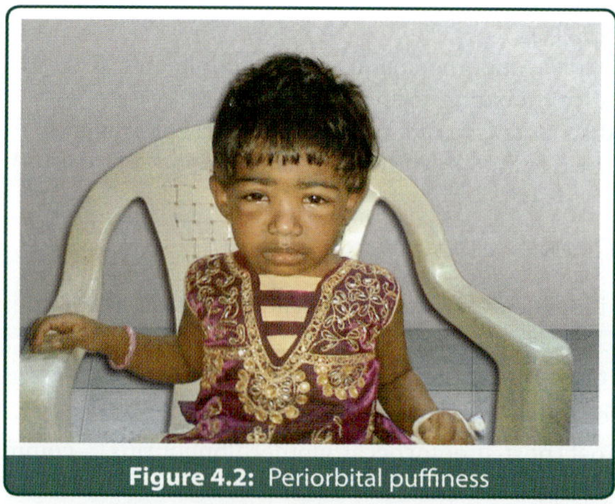

Figure 4.2: Periorbital puffiness

Anthropometry

- Height
- Weight
- Head circumference
- Chest circumference.

SYSTEMIC EXAMINATION

Abdomen- R/o Hepatosplenomegaly
Palpate for kidney
Look for renal angle tenderness
Suprapubic tenderness (cystitis)
Free fluid

CVS
RS – Pleural effusion (nephrotic syndrome)
CNS

DIAGNOSIS

- **AGN**
- **Nephrotic syndrome**

Viva Questions

Urine in AGN is cola colored. Why? (Fig. 4.3)

'**Acid hematin'** is produces the color.

Urine color in Nephrotic Syndrome:

1. White/straw color
2. Gets frothy in the container (due to increased protein)
3. Decreased/normal output

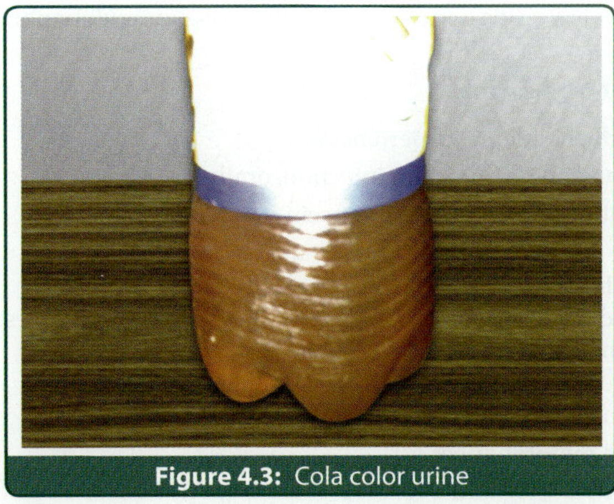

Figure 4.3: Cola color urine

Differences between edema in

Acute glomerulonephritis	*Nephrotic syndrome*
• Turgid	• Soft
• Does not pit easily	• Pits readily

ACUTE GLOMERULONEPHRITIS (AGN)

- Rapid onset
- Minimal edema (puffiness of face periorbital edema)
- Oliguria
- H/O Preceding sore throat (or) skin infections (or) scabies
- Increased BP
- Hematuria
- No history of similar episodes
- Anemia.

Investigations

- Hematuria
- Renal function test/urine C/S
- To prove AGN/to exclude nephrotic syndrome

1. **Urine:** Macroscopic : Less quantity/high-colored urine(cola colored)
   Microscopic: RBC casts + Granular hyaline casts + Bacteria (UTI)
   Urinary protein: Not of much rise (1+)
2. **Serum**: Urea/creatinine levels: Increased depending upon renal function alteration
3. **Chest X-ray**: Hypervolemia can lead to pulmonary congestion, cardiomegaly
4. **Blood**: Protein, TC, DC, ESR, serum cholesterol
5. **ASO tirte:** Antihyaluronidase, AntiDNAse units increased
6. **Throat culture**
7. **C3 level decreased** : By 6 weeks, it will be normal if not by 6 months—R/O systems conditions; polyarteritis nodosa or other form of glomerulonephritis.

Management of AGN

1. **Bed rest**: Reduces edema/hypertension
2. **Penicillin**: 50,000-1lac units IM injection/orally
   (or) amoxicillin/ampicillin/erythromycin (for 10 days)
3. **Diet**:
   - No added salt
   - Fluids and salt restriction (sodium: 0.5 g/day—amount adding salt in separator)
   - Solids can be taken unlimited
   - Fruit juices/tender coconuts to be avoided
   - Sweet can be given (payasam, sweet pongal)
4. **Input-output maintenance:**
   - **1st day Input**: 20 mL/kg/day

Insensible water loss = 400 mL

- **2nd day Input**: Calculate the total urine output on day I; add 400 mL with this (output + 400 mL) amount.

Example: 800 mL is output on day 1

Input 2nd day: 800 + 400 = 1200 mL fluid today

Replaced:

- Insensible loss by
  10% Dextrose
- **Urine output by**
  50%—normal saline
  50%—dextrose 10%

5. **Control of blood pressure:**
   >90 mm Hg diastolic, give
   - Sublingual nifedipine—0.01 mg/kg/day
   - Monitor ½ hourly for first 2 hours then 8th hourly (or) twice daily
   - BP ≤90 mm Hg: Give oral—nifedipine/hydralazine/atenolol

   Ask mother to keep head low position(since hypotension is frequent)
6. **Hypertensive crisis:**
   1st alpha methyldopa: 5–10 mg/kg IV drip
   Give Na^+—**Nitroprusside** = 0.5–8 µg/kg IV infusion
   Diazoxide = 5 mg/kg
   Nifedipine sublingual 300–500 mg/kg.

Monitor weight regularly: Loss should be an 0.5% of actual body weight every day

- Diuretics: Frusemide: 2 mg/kg/BW
- Indication:
  - Severe edema
  - Pulmonary congestion
  - Left ventricular failure.

Prognosis: Excellent in AGN

- Resolve in 2 weeks
- If not, renal biopsy to review the diagnosis
- Recurrence is rare
  - Macroscopic hematuria disappears by 2–3 weeks
  - Microscopic hematuria disappears by 6 months–1 year.

Complications

1. Hypertensive encephalopathy
2. Left ventricular failure; pulmonary edema
3. Electrolyte disturbances
4. RPGN—very rarely needs dialysis
5. Chronic renal failure.

Why renal edema is over face first?

1. Loose areola tissue
2. Patients are ambulant

What is cause of anemia?

1. Dilutional
2. Hematuria

Causes of palpable kidney?

1. Hydronephrosis
2. Wilm's tumor
3. Polycystic kidney disease

What should be monitored before giving Frusemide?

- Blood urea
- Serum creatinine
- In case of increased blood urea when diuretics given because of uremia leads to encephalopathy, DIC

NEPHROTIC SYNDROME

- Young children (2–6 years)
- Insidious onset
- Massive edema/ascites; pleural effusion and hydrocele
- H/O Previous similar episodes (recurrence)
- H/O Steroid therapy
- H/O Normal/high-colored urine with normal quantity
- No H/O hematuria
- No hypertension
- In examination also, BP normal.

Investigations

- To diagnose protein in urine/ to include hematuria
- To diagnose blood protein level
- To diagnose cholesterol.

1. Urine Examination: Macroscopic—normal quantity/normal or high-colored
   Microscopic—no hematuria (hyaline, waxy casts)
   24 hour urine protein—>0.1 g/kg/h—heavy proteinuria

   Tests
   1. Heat coagulation test
   2. Sulfosalicylic acid test
   3. Albustix test
   4. Esbach Albuminometer

   WBC cast—pyelonephritis
   RBC morphology—altered when seen in phase contrast

   To diagnose hypoproteinemia:
   1. Serum albumin (N: 3.5–5 g/dL)
   2. A:G ratio (normal globulin: 1.5–3.5 g/dL)
   3. Serum: Protein/creatinine ratio (N: <0.3)

   4. Blood urea (N:20–40 mg/dL)
   5. Serum creatinine (N: 0.1 to 0.5 mg/dL)
   6. Electrophoresis mobility pattern
2. Serum: Total protein decreased
   Albumin level <2.5 g/dL
   Abumin: Globulin ratio reversed
3. Serum: Creatinine, protein ratio
   Normal: 0.7–1.5 mg/100 mL
   More than 3.5 = Nephrotic syndrome
4. Plasma urea, creatinine, elevated
5. Serum cholesterol: Elevated >200–220 mg%
   Proteinuria: >50mg/kg/day
6. Chest X-ray/mantoux: To R/O TB; because TB will flare up on steroid therapy
7. Serum electrolytes
8. Electrophoretic motility pattern: Albumin decreased, decreased α_2 globulin; AG reversal

Management (Figs 4.4 and 4.5)

Bed Rest

Furosemide: 1 mg/kg BW (tds or BD) to relieve edema with sodium, potassium and calcium supplements.

1. Monitor electrolytes
2. Diet/fluid correction: Refer AGN
3. Give protein such diet: Milk/white of egg
4. Treat other infections:
   - Pneumococcal pneumonia
   - Pneumococcal pneumonitis
5. Treat the TB
6. Steroid therapy: 2 mg/kg BW/day—for 6 weeks
   If there is nil proteinuria for 3 days after therapy, Taper the dose

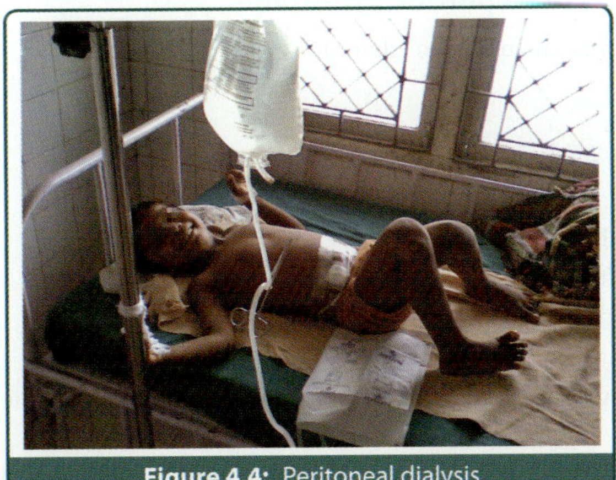

Figure 4.4: Peritoneal dialysis

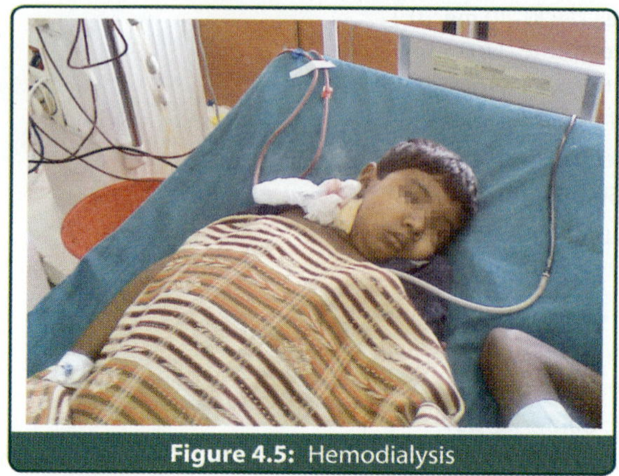

Figure 4.5: Hemodialysis

- 1.5 mg/kg—next 4 weeks
- 1 mg/kg—next 4 weeks
- 0.5 mg/kg—next 4 weeks and stop drug

7. Prophylactic antibiotics
8. Relapse: Common—

   Steroids - 2 mg/kg/day for 10–14 weeks

   Taper the dose if there is nil proteinuria for 3 days successively.

   1.5/1/0.5 mg/kg for 4 weeks successively.

   Frequent relapses:
   - Give above treat with above 0.5 mg/kg—alternate days for 1 year
   - More than 4 episodes/1 year
9. **Steroid resistant cases:**
   - Review by renal biopsy

   Treatment:
   - Cyclophosphamide
   - Cyclosporin
   - Methotrexate.

Complications of Nephrotic Syndrome

- Electrolyte imbalance (due to edema)
- Peritonitis
- Pneumonitis
- Cellulitis
- Meningitis
- Thromboembolic manifests
- Acute renal failure.

Prognosis

- Child will have no residual dysfunction after 2nd decade up to which, relapses may occur
- Child may become fertile (except when cyclophosphamide or chlorambucil—sterile).

PROTEINURIA

Normal: 150 mg/24 h
Mild: 0.5 g/24 h
Moderate: 0.5–2 g/24 h
Massive: >2 g/24 h

- Hypoproteinemia is due to proteinuria >2g/24h
- Hematuria: (h/o)
  Proximal—Urethritis(RBC morphology not altered)
  Terminal—Cystitis
  - Schistosomiasis
  - Calculi

  Throughout - AGN (altered RBC morphology)
- DD—red urine:
  1. Hematuria
  2. Hemoglobinopathies
  3. Rifampicin
  4. Beet root
  5. Coloring dyes
  6. Porphyrias
  7. Newborn.

Causes of Hematuria

- AGN
- Nephrotic syndrome (H/O fever, infection)
- Rent calculi (H/O abdominal pain)
- Bleeding diathesis (H/O purpuric spots)
- Cystitis, UTI, hemangiomas
- **Drugs**: Sulfonamides, aspirin, cyclophosphamide.

Macroscopic Hematuria

Coca or coffee-colored urine
Frank blood-extraglomerular.

Microscopic Hematuria

>2 RBC/HPF - uncentrifuged urine
>5 RBC/ HP - centrifuged urine.

Tests to Detect Proteinuria

1+ : 30 mg/dL
2+ : 200 mg/dL
3+ : 300 mg/dL
4+ : 2000 mg/dL

Heat Coagulation Test

- Fill 2/3 of test tube with the sample
- Heat the upper part, opalescence is formed

- Add a few drops of (acetic acid-glacial)
  - Disappears: Phosphate +
  - Persists: Protein.

Sulfosalicylic Acid Test

- To 5 mL sample, add 5 drops of 10% sulfosalicylic acid (white precipitate formed).

ACUTE STREPTOCOCCAL GLOMERULONEPHRITIS

Most common cause of hematuria: IgA nephropathy

1. Characterized by: Sudden onset of
   1. Acute hematuria
   2. Edema
   3. Hypertension
   4. Final

Etiology and Epidemiology

Follows infection of throat/skin
With certain nephritogenic strains of Group A beta-hemolytic streptococci

- Cold weather - AGN follow streptococcal pharyngitis
- Warm weather - AGN follows skin infections and pyoderma
- Epidemics of nephritis have been associated with serotype 12 (throat) also serotype 4 and serotype 49 (skin)

AGN follows:
Respiratory infection in 2–3 weeks
Skin infection in 4–6 weeks

Pathology:

- kidneys symmetrically enlarged
- Light microscopy - all glomeruli enlarged
  - Relatively blood less
  - Diffuse mesangial cell proliferation
  - Increase in mesangial matrix
- Polymorphonuclear leukocytes are common (early stages)
- Crescents (severe cases).

Immunofluorescence

- 'Lumpy-bumpy deposits' of immunoglobin
- Deposits of immunoglobulin and complex on GBM and mesangium.

Electron Microscopy

Electron dense deposits (HUMPS) on the epithelial side of GBM (Glomerular basement membrane).

Pathogenesis

- Decreased serum complement (C3) level
- Suggests immune complex-mediated.

Clinical Features

1. >3 years age (rare before 3 years)
2. H/O Streptococcal infection 1–2 week before

C/O Hematuria(cola-colored urine)
Edema (due to salt and water retention)
Hypertension
Oliguria

Severe cases - Encephalopathy (c/o-convulsions)
—Congestive heart failure

Non-specific symptom:

- Malaise
- Lethargy
- Flank pain
- Fever

Acute phase resolves in/month urinary abnormalities persist > 1 year.

Diagnosis

Urinalysis

- Red blood cells
- Red cell casts +
- Proteinuria
- Polymorphonuclear leukocytes → Infection.

Blood

Normochromic and normocytic anemia—mild (due to hemodilution low grade hemolysis).

Serum C3

Decreased.

Chest X-ray

Increased vascular markings (hypovolemia).

USG finding in AGN

Cortex and medulla will be of different echo density normally. But in AGN both cortex and medulla have same gradient.

Confirmation

Evidence of streptococcal infection:

1. Positive throat culture - shows carrier state
2. Elevated ASO titer - not specific
   (Normal: 200 Todd units)
3. Best—antibody titer to DNAse B antigen

4. Alternative:
   "Streptozyme Test"
   Side agglutination test that detects antibodies to:
   i. Streptolysin O
   ii. DNAse B
   iii. Hyaluronidase
   iv. Streptokinase
   v. NADase.

Renal Biopsy

Not indicated in

i. A child with AGN
ii. Evidence of recent streptococcal infection
iii. Low C3 level
iv. Clinical diagnosis evident of AGN

Indicated to exclude

i. SLE
ii. Acute exacerbation of chronic glomerulonephritis

Renal biopsy is not needed if the patient has the following features:

- Decreased C3 level
- Evidence of streptococcal infection
- Clinical diagnosis of AGN

Considerations for Renal Biopsy

1. Development of ARF
2. Development of nephrotic syndrome
3. Absent evidence of streptococcal infection
4. Absence of hypocomplementemia, i.e. no decrease in C3 level
5. Low C3 for more than 3 months
6. Persistent hematuria
7. Persistent proteinuria
8. Diminished renal function

Other Organisms Causing AGN

1. Coagulate +/- staphylococci
2. Streptococcus pneumonia
3. Gram-negative bacteria
4. Fungal/Rickettsial/Viral.

Complications

1. Acute Renal future
2. Volume overload
3. Circulatory congestion
4. Hypertension

5. Hyperkalemia
6. Hyperphosphatemia
7. Hypocalcemia/natremia
8. Acidosis
9. Seizures
10. Uremia: Encephalopathy

Prevention

- Early systemic antibiotic therapy to skin/throat infections
- Screening family members/treating if positive for culture.

Prognosis

- Complete recovery—95% cases
- In 5% cases—glomerular hyalinization and chronic renal insufficiency.

Differential Diagnosis for Hematuria (Acute Glomerulonephritis)

I. Glomerular Disease

1. Recurrent gross hematuria syndrome
   IgA nephropathy
   Idiopathic (benign familial) hypercalciuric calciuria
   Alport's (+deafness)
2. Acute post-streptococcal GN
3. MPGN/RPGN
4. SLE
5. Goodpasture's disease (+ hemoptysis)
6. Hemolytic uremic syndrome
7. Membranous glomerulopathy

II. Infection

- Bacterial
- Tuberculosis
- Viral

III. Hematologic

- Coagulopathies
- Thrombocytopenia
- Sickle cell disease
- Renal vein thrombosis

IV. Stones/hypercalciuria

V. Exercise

VI. Drugs

VII. Anatomic abnormalities

- Congenital anomalies
- Trauma
- PC kidney (polycystic)
- Vascular anomalies
- Tumor

NEPHROTIC SYNDROME

1. **Characteristic Features:**
   - Proteinuria
   - Hypoproteinemia
   - Edema
   - Hyperlipidemia
2. **Etiology:**
   - 90%: Idiopathic:
     Minimal change disease—80%
     Mesangial proliferation—15%
     Focal sclerosis—10%
   - 10%—some form of glomerulonephritis
     Membranous MPGN (common)

Pathophysiology

1. Proteinuria:

   Underlying pathogenetic abnormality due to increased capillary wall permeability. Increased glomerular capillary wall permeability.
   i. Loss of negatively charged glycoproteins in the capillary wall
   ii. Focal segmental glomerulosclerosis (FSGS)
   FSGS: Plasma factor produced by lymphocytes which increase the glomerular permeability
   * Protein loss >2g/24 h
   (primarily albumin)
   Edema appears when—serum albumin <2.5 g/dL
2. Edema:

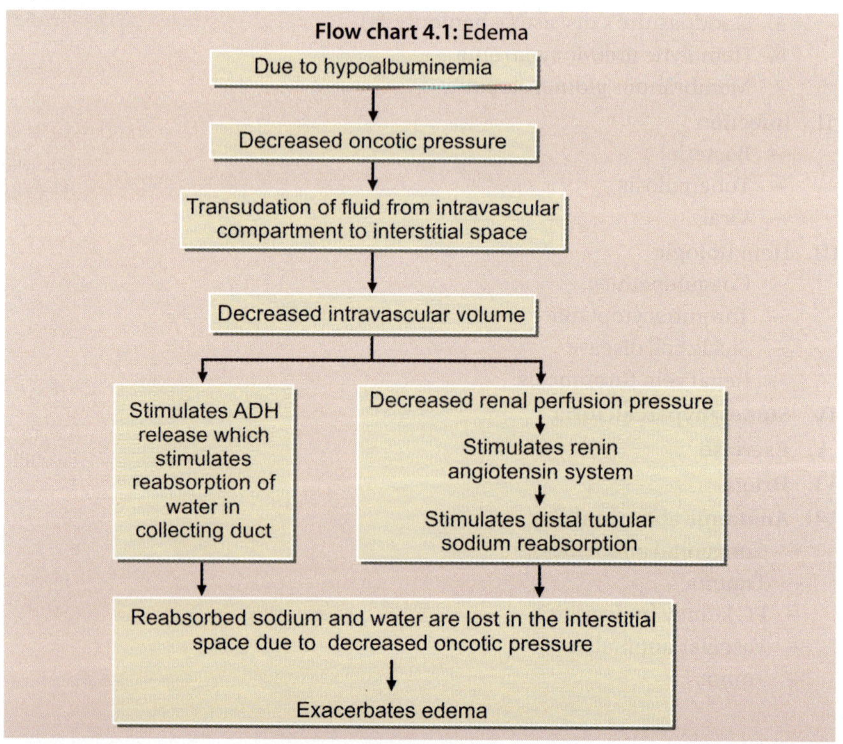

i. **Hypothesis:**

Intrarenal deficit in sodium and water excretion

Presence of circulating agent increases capillary wall permeability throughout body and kidney.

3. **Hyperlipidemia:**
   1. Hypoproteinemia: Generalized protein synthesis including lipoproteins
   2. Lipid catabolism decreased due to reduced plasma levels of lipoprotein lipase (enzyme that is essential for removing lipids from plasma)

   Increased serum cholesterol/serum thyroglobulin and serum lipoprotein).

IDIOPATHIC NEPHROTIC SYNDROME

Accounts for 90% nephrosis in children.

Etiology

1. Immunologic-mediated (but evidence of classic mechanism of immunologic injury is lacking)
2. IgE mediated
3. Abnormality in thymus (T-Cell) lymphocyte function.

Pathology

Three morphological patterns:

Minimal change disease (85%)	*Mesangial proliferation group (5%)*	*Focal sclerosis lesion (10%)*
Glomeruli appear normal or show a minimal increase in mesangial cells and matrix	Diffuse increases in mesangial cells and matrix	Majority appear normal or show mesangial proliferation; others close to medulla show segmental scarring in one or more lobules (similar scarring is seen in HIV infection, vesicoureteric reflux and intravenous heroine use)
Electron microscopy. Relaxation of epithelial cell foot process	Mesangial deposits of IgM and C3	
95% children responds to steroids	50–60% responds to steroids	**Salient pathological features of FSGS:** • Scarring • End stage renal failure (by involving all glomeruli) • 20% respond to corticosteroids or cytotoxic drugs • Recur in transplanted kidney

Clinical Manifestation

Boys:Girls = 2:1
Age group = 2–6 years
(also reported earlier than 1 year and in adults)

- Apparent upper respiratory tract infection: Initial episode and subsequent relapses
- Edema
  - Initially around eyes
  - Lower extremities (pitting type)
  - Later becomes generalized
- Generalized edema- associated weight gain, pleural effusion, ascites and declining urine output
- Edema accumulate in dependent sites
- H/O Shift from face and back to abdomen and leg.

H/O Anorexia
Abdominal pain
Diarrhea.

Investigation

Urinalysis:

- +3 or +4 proteinuria
- Microscopic hematuria
- Low creatinine clearance
  (due to diminished renal perfusion resulting from contraction of the intravascular volume)
- Protein excretion: >2g/24h
- Serum values:
  - Serum cholesterol—increased
  - Serum triglycerides—increased
  - Serum albumin—decreased
  - Serum calcium—decreased
- Complement C3 level—normal
  - In AGN C3 decreased upto 6 weeks.

Complications

1. Infections:
   - Immunoglobulin levels
   - Edema fluid acts as a culture medium
   - Protein deficiency
   - Decreased bactericidal activity of leukocytes
   - Immunosuppressive therapy (e.g. cyclophosphamide)
   - Perfusion of spleen (due to hypovolemia)
   - Urinary loss of a complement (Properdin factor B) that opsonizes certain bacteria
   - Spontaneous peritonitis (most frequent)—caused by streptococcal pneumonia
   - Sepsis
   - Cellulitis
   - Pneumonia
   - UTI

Viva: What vaccine should be given to the patients having nephrosis (during remittent phase)

'Polyvalent pneumococcal vaccine'

Viva: In the presence of corticosteroid therapy:

Fever and other physical findings are minimal.

Therefore, start antibiotic therapy with high index of suspicion.

2. Arterial/Venous Thrombosis:
   - Renal, pulmonary, cerebral vein thrombosis (Fig. 4.6)
   - Elevated plasma level of certain coagulation factors
   - In history of fibrinolysis
   - Decreased plasma level of anti-thrombin III
   - Increased platelet aggregation
   - Deficiency of coagulation factors: IX, XI and XII
   - Reduced serum level of vitamin D:
   - ARF: Rapid diuresis/acute gastroenteritis aggravate hypovolemia.

Treatment

General Measures to Treat Edema

1. Diet: High protein and low salt

   'no added salt'

   Restriction of fluid (severe edema)

   Protein rich diet- eggs
2. Diuretics:

   Mild—salt restriction/frusemide small doses

   Massive with ascites—Furosemide (3–5 mg/kg) with spironolactone and hydrochlorothiazide

   If serum albumin level is less than 1 g/dL with hypovolemia: Human albumin IV (0.5–1 g/kg) followed by intravenous furosemide (2–3 mg/kg)
3. Prophylaxis to infection.

Remission

Current policy: (APN Regimen)

- 6 weeks divided doses—prednisolone 2 mg/kg/day (2–3 divided)
- Next 6 weeks single morning dose—prednisolone 1–5 mg/kg/day.

Care taken:

i. Give antacids

ii. Monitor BP

To Prevent Relapse

Infrequent: 3 or less/per year
Frequent: 4 or more/per year

Treatment: For Infrequent relapse
Prednisolone: 2 mg/kg/day until urine becomes protein-free for 3 days followed by (if free) **Prednisolone:** 1.5 mg/kg/day for 4 weeks.

Treatment: Plan for frequent relapse
Mode 1: (Steroids)

- Alternate day prednisolone: 9–12 months (0.3–0.7 mg/kg for 9–12 months)

Mode 2:
Levamisole (2–2.5 mg/kg) daily
Immunomodulant + prednisolone (1.5 mg/kg) on alternate days

Mode 3: Alkylating agents
Cyclophosphamide (2 mg/kg) + prednisolone as above—both on alternate days

Side effect

- Hemorrhagic cystitis
- Gonadal toxicity
- Leukopenia (monitor WBC)
- Vomiting
- Alopecia.

To prevent cystitis:

1. Liberal fluid
2. Give the dose early morning (it is a contact poison, so it can be excreted all over the day)
3. 'Mesna' can be given

Mode 4: Cyclosporin A: 5 mg/kg/day + prednisolone as above on alternate days 1–3 years

Side effect:

- Hypertension
- Hirsuitism
- Gum hyperplasia
- Nephro toxic.

End Stage Renal Failure

Renal Transplant

What is:

1. **Remission:** Clinical/urine normal in 8 weeks of steroid treatment
2. **Resistant:** Not responds in 8 weeks (still proteniuria +)
3. **Steroid dependence**: Becomes positive while tapering the dose or while switching from continuous 6 weeks to alternate 6 weeks
4. **Relapse**: Becomes positive >3 weeks after completion of course

Glomerulonephritis (Fig. 4.7)

Nephrotic syndrome may develop during the course of:

- Membranous (Fig. 4.6)
- MPGN
- Post-streptococcal
- Lupus (SLE) (Figs 4.8A and B)
- Chronic infection malaria and schistosomiasis
- Henoch-Schönlein purpura.

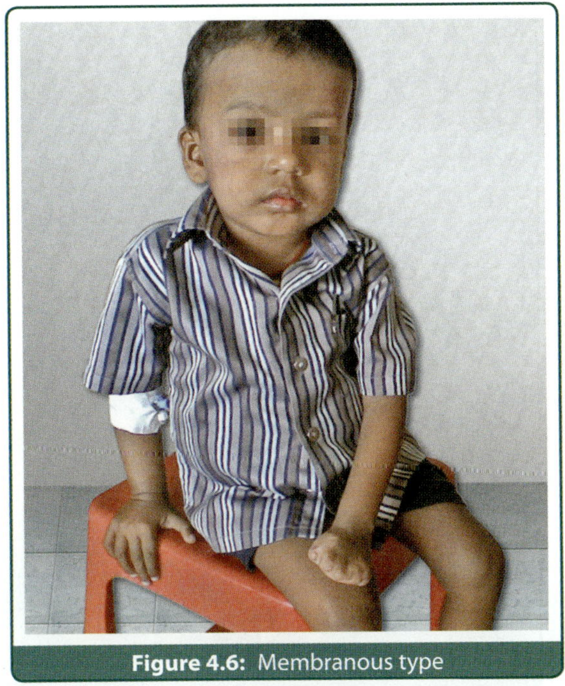

Figure 4.6: Membranous type

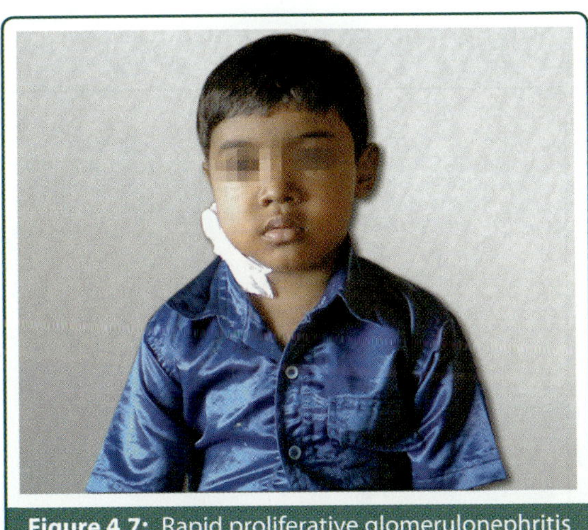

Figure 4.7: Rapid proliferative glomerulonephritis

Tumors

- Mediated by immune complexes composed of tumor antigens and tumor-specific antibodies
  - Hodgkin's lymphoma: Minimal change disease, membranous type
  - May be because the tumor produces a lymphokine that increases glomerular capillary wall permeability.

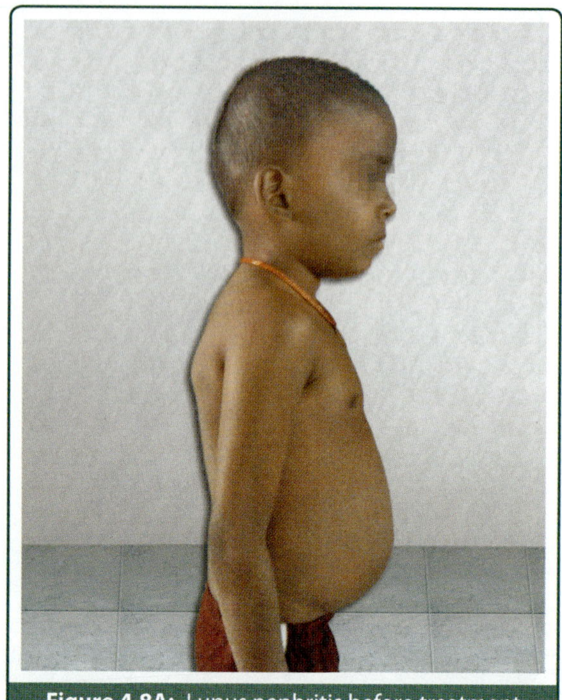

Figure 4.8A: Lupus nephritis before treatment

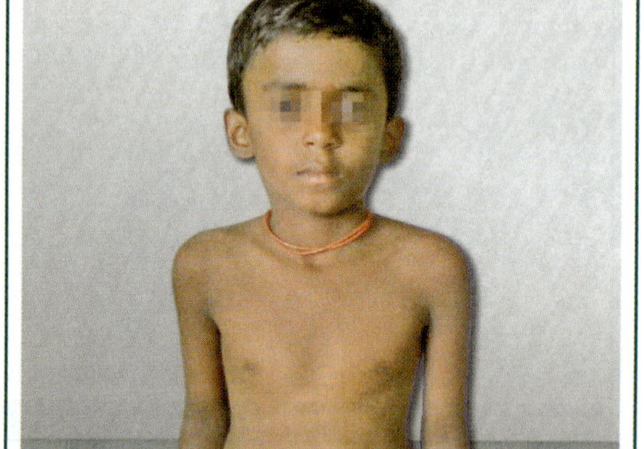

Figure 4.8B: Lupus after treatment

Drugs

Histologic picture of:

- Membranous Glomerulopathy:
  - Penicillamine
  - NSAIDS
  - Mercury
- Minimal change disease:
  - Probenecid
  - Ethosuximide
  - Lithium: Side effect—Ebstein's anomaly, tricuspid atresia
- Proliferative glomerulonephritis (Fig. 4.8):
  - Procainamide
  - Phenytoin
  - Chlorpropamide
  - Trimethadione.

Congenital Nephrotic Syndrome

- Nephrotic syndrome is rare during first 3 years of life
- Acute glomerulonephritis will never occur in < 3 years
- Causes for nephrotic syndrome during first 6 months:
  - Congenital NS
  - Congenital infection (syphilis, toxoplasmosis, CMV)
  - Diffuse mesangial sclerosis of unknown cause

Drash Syndrome

- Nephropathy
- Wilm's tumor
- Genital abnormalities

Congenital Nephrotic Syndrome (Finnish Type)

- Autosomal recessive
- Long arm chromosome 19
- Major pathologic feature—dilatation of proximal convoluted tubules
- Pathogenesis: Decrease in number of heparin sulfate rich anionic sites in GBM.

Other clinical features include:

- Prematurity
- Enlarged placenta
- Respiratory distress
- Separation of cranial sutures

Death by age of 5 years - Infection or renal failure
Diagnosis can be made antenatal by measuring alpha fetoprotein level at 16–20 weeks gestation

Treatment: Captopril/indomethacin/unilateral nephrectomy
Ultimate - kidney transplant
Corticosteroids/immunosuppressants—no value.

Do for edematous face:

- Generalized anasarca
- Decreased oncotic pressure
- CCF
- Kwashiorkor
- Anemia
- Angioneurotic edema
- Myxedema
- Cushingoid feature
- Lawrence-Moon-Biedl syndrome

Head to Foot Examination (To make DD)
Head

- Increased ICT
- Wide open sutures (congenital nephrotic syndrome)
- Dull facies (hypothyroidism)

Face

- Delayed eruption of teeth (R/O: Hypothyroidism)
- Signs of vitamin deficiency (R/O: Kwashiorkor)

Neck

- Raised JVP (CCF)
- Lymphadenitis

Values to be known:

1. Serum:
   Urea: 20 mg/dL
   Creatinine: 0.2–0.5 mg/dL
   Creatinine clearance: 80–120 mL/mt/1.73 m^2
   Serum cholesterol: <200 mg/dL
   (>220 mg/dL = hypercholesterolemia)
2. Urine:
   i. Proteinuria: Normal: <150 mg/24 h
      Mild: 0.5 g/24 h
      Moderate: 0.5–2 g/24 h
      Massive: >2 g/24 h
      (Or)
   ii. Proteinuria: >50 mg/kg/day (>0.5 g/day)
   iii. 24 hour urine protein: >0.1 g/kg/h/day
   iv. Heat coagulation test:
      1+ : 30 mg/dL – you can read
      2+ : 200 mg/dL
      3+ : 300 mg/dL – can't read hack lines
      4+ : 200 mg/dL
3. Serum:
   Albumin: <2.5 g/dL (hypoalbuminemia)
   Serum protein/creatinine: Normal: <0.3
   AGN: 0.3–3
   NS: >3
4. Oliguria: <1 mL/kg/h

What is the Meaning of

Remission: Clinical/urine—Normal in 8 weeks
In <4 weeks: Early responder
> 4 weeks: Late responder
Resistant: Not responds in still 8 weeks
Dependence: Clinically, urine protein becomes positive while tapering or in < 3 weeks
Relapse: Clinically, urine protein becomes positive in > 3 weeks

OP Ghai:

- Frequent relapse: 4 or more frequent per year (≥4/year)
- Infrequent relapse: 3 or less infrequent (≤3/year)

Selective proteinuria:
Only albumin lost
For example, Minimal change disease (nephrotic syndrome).

Proteins Lost in Nephrotic Syndrome

1. Albumin
2. Transferrin
3. Anti-thrombin III
4. Thyroxine-binding globulin
5. Cholecalciferol protein
6. Metal-binding proteins.

CASE 5 Cardiovascular System

[PDA, TOF, ASD, VSD, RHD (MS, MR, AS)]

Incidence of congenital heart disease:
General population incidence: 6–8%

- ASD and PDA: 6–8% each
- TOF: 5–10%
- VSD: 15–20%

HISTORY TAKING

Eight-month-old 2nd child born of a non-consanguineous marriage was brought to the hospital by the mother whose reliability is good with presenting

C/O:

- Breathlessness
- Recurrent respiratory tract infection (RTI) > 6 years
- Easy: Fatigability
- Swelling in legs/all over body
- Palpitation
- Syncope
- Feeding difficulties
- Failure to thrive
- Joint pain with swelling.

Other relevant histories:

- H/O Symptoms from birth/after how long
- H/O Cyanosis
- H/O Squatting
- H/O Recurrent lower respiratory track infection (LRTI)
  - H/O Chest retraction
  - H/O Tachypnea
  - H/O Feeding difficulty
- H/O Frequent hospitalization
- H/O Joint pain, swelling, fever
- H/O Sore throat
- H/O PND/orthopnea
- H/O Feeding difficulties
- H/O Profuse sweating while feeding
- H/O Protracted fever (IE)
- H/O Right hypochondrial pain
- H/O CCF in infants (On feeding, takes only inadequate amount and so feels hungry and cries for feeds → and again feeding takes only inadequate amount and this cycle continues).

Past History

- H/O Similar episodes before
- H/O RTI recurrent/how many times
- H/O Any continuous medication for CCF
- H/O Any previous hospitalization
- H/O Any surgery
- H/O Exanthematous illness in mother (Rubella)
- H/O TB
- H/O Neurological deficit
- H/O Bleeding tendencies

  (In cyanotic spells, there will be neurological deficit and bleeding tendencies).

Antenatal History

TORCH infection (fever with rash)
Rubella: PDA(most common), coarctation of aorta, VSD, pulmonary stenosis (H/O posterior auricular node)
Mumps: Endocarditis

H/O Serial abortions: (3, 5, 7, 9 months)—syphilis
(Note: Reverse order: 1st child escapes, 2nd child at 9th month, next at 7 months, 5 months in case of RH incompatibility)

H/O Drug intake:

- T : Thalidomide; trimetazidine—TOF
- H : Hydantoin
- A : Alcohol
- L : Lithium
- I : Iodine
- D : Dextroamphetamine
- O : Oestrogens (OCP)
- M : Methotrexate
- I : Irradiation, indomethacin
- D : Valproate
- E : Epileptic (antiepileptic drugs)

H/O maternal illness: Diabetes—asymmetrical septal HT

- Obstetric cardiomyopathy
- VSD
- ASD
- TGA.

Natal History

Term/preterm:

- Preterm: PDA will persist for a longer time i.e., we can wait for 1 year, no need to give indomethacin if symptomatic
- Full-term: PDA closes by 10–21 days
- If PDA persists, give indomethacin

- H/O cyanosis at birth (tricuspid atresia, transposition of great arteries)
- H/O birth asphyxia (hypoxia—persistent PDA)
- H/O birth at high altitudes (persistent PDA).

Postnatal History

- H/O Breastfeeding
- H/O Tachypnea, dyspnea
- H/O Hospitalization after birth—cause, duration, treatment rendered
- H/O Paucity of movements
- H/O Cyanosis, convulsions, jaundice, respiratory distress, umbilical sepsis
- H/O Delayed passage of meconium (normally passed in 24 hours)—cystic fibrosis.

Development History

Diet History

Family History

- H/O similar illness in the siblings
- H/O any other family members
- H/O maternal diabetes: (TGA, hypoplastic heart)
- H/O consanguineous marriage (may have chromosomal anomalies) (Down's syndrome—PDA, ASD).

GENERAL EXAMINATION

- Anemia
- Cyanosis (Fig. 5.1)
- Clubbing (Fig. 5.2)
- Pedal edema
- Jaundice
- Lymphadenopathy
- Nutritional status
- Any vitamin deficiency
- Any focal sepsis (dental and oral examination for dental caries)
- Features of chromosomal anomalies: Down's syndrome
- Congenital abnormalities.

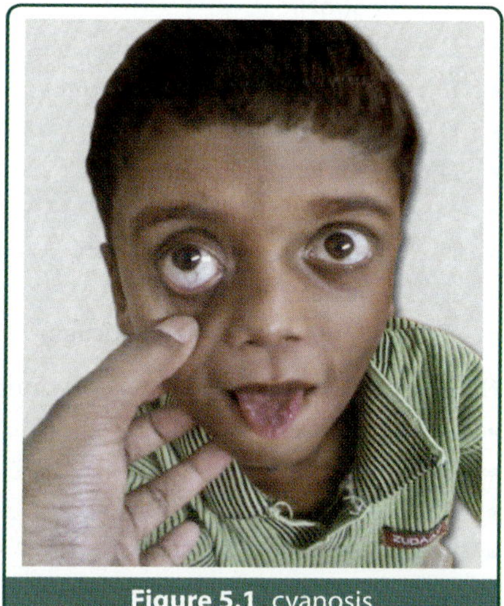

Figure 5.1 cyanosis

Markers of CVS diseases:

- Microcephaly
- Mangolian slant
- Hypertelorism (increased interpupillary distance)
- Low set ears
- Polydactyly (PDA—female child)
- Cleft palate/lip (septal defect)
- Limb defects (ASD with bone deformity) (Holt Oram Syndrome).

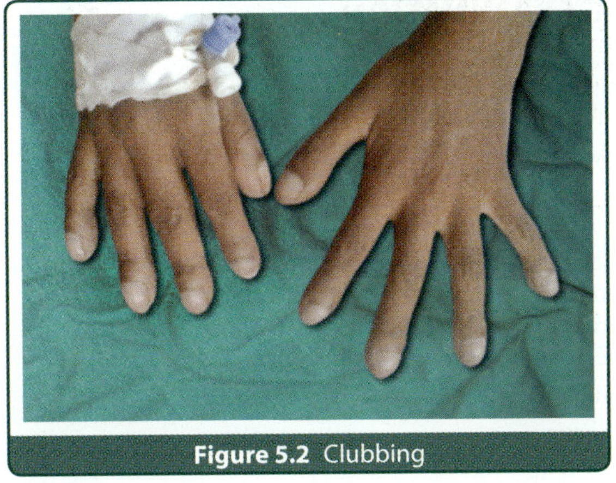

Figure 5.2 Clubbing

Anti-Mongoloid slant:
(Pneumonic-Noon Cat TT)

- Noonan syndrome
- Cat cry syndrome
- Turner syndrome
- Trisomy 17–18
- Treacher Collins syndrome.

Mongoloid slant:
(slanting of eyes in the shape of letter "M")

- Down's syndrome
- Ectodermal dysplasia
- Prader-Willi syndrome.

Signs of rheumatic fever:

- Erythema marginatum
- Subcutaneous nodules
- Joint swelling
- Chorea

Peripheral signs of infective endocarditis:

- Persistent fever (7–10 days)
- Anemia
- Osler's nodes (painful)
- Janeway lesions (painless)
- Changing murmurs (varying quality)

- spleen +
- splinter hemorrhages
- Roth spots
- Hematuria
- clubbing

Vital Sign

- Pulse rate
- Blood pressure
- Temperature
- Respiratory rate.

Anthropometric measures: (See details in Chapter 1)

SYSTEMIC EXAMINATION

Inspection

- JVP
- Apical impulse
- Trachea
- Pulsations
  - Supraclavicular: Thyroid pulsation, aneurysm of arch of aorta, aortic regurgitation
  - Suprasternal: Right atrial enlargement
  - Epigastric: Right ventricular hypertrophy
- Precordial bulge
- Parasternal heave.

Palpation

- Measures JVP
- Apical impulse: Pulse and character
- Parasternal heave
- Palpable sounds
- Palpable murmur (thrill)
- Confirm trachea.

Percussion

- Some examiners ask to percuss the borders.

Auscultation

Four areas (Mitral/tricuspid/pulmonary/aortic)

- Infraclavicular: (PDA) left 1st intercostal space—**Gibson's area**
- 2nd aortic area: (ERB's area) Aortic regurgitation—left 3rd ICS
- Left 3rd and 4th space (**Rogers Area**)—VSD
- Back: Interscapular—Suzman's sign-coarctation

Examination of Other Systems

- CNS
- RS
- Abdomen.

Nada's Criteria

Major criteria:
- Congestive cardiac failure
- Cyanosis
- Diastolic murmur
- Systolic murmur (>Grade 3)

Minor criteria
- Abnormal X-ray
- Abnormal ECG
- Abnormal Sound S_2
- Abnormal BP

Diagnosis

Eight-year-old—is a case of acyanotic congenital heart disease probably VSD, with left to right shunt and PEM and patient not in feature with sinus rhythm and no PHT.

Investigations

- Blood: Hemoglobin%, TC, DC and ESR
- Chest X-ray/urine RBC
- Echo: Diagnosis can be confirmed
- ECG
- Cardiac catheterization = pulmonary HTN.

MANAGEMENT

- Rx anemia
- Rx IE
- Rx CCF
- Rx infections
- Feeding through IV/nasogastric tube
- Fluid intake-output chart
- Finally, surgical management.

VENTRICULAR SEPTAL DEFECT (FIG. 5.3)

The VSD is a defect in the ventricular septum either single or multiple either in membranous or muscular part resulting in L → R or R → L shunt.

History Taking

C/O: Recurrent RTI

- Diagnosed by a private practitioners
- Tachypnea/dyspnea
- Poor weight gain

G/E. built (poor weight gain)
Pallor (R/O cause of breathlessness)
Cyanosis (Reversal of shunt)
Eye: congenital cataract, congenital rubella syndrome

Facies:

- Elfin facies: Supravalvular AS
- Down's endocardial cushion defect
- Mitral facies: MS (malar flush and peripheral cyanosis)
- Cyanotic facies

Ears: Low set
Palate: Cleft palate
Neck: Web neck, short neck, low hair line (below C5)

- Dyspnea
- Tachypnea
- Subcostal retraction
- Acutely ill.

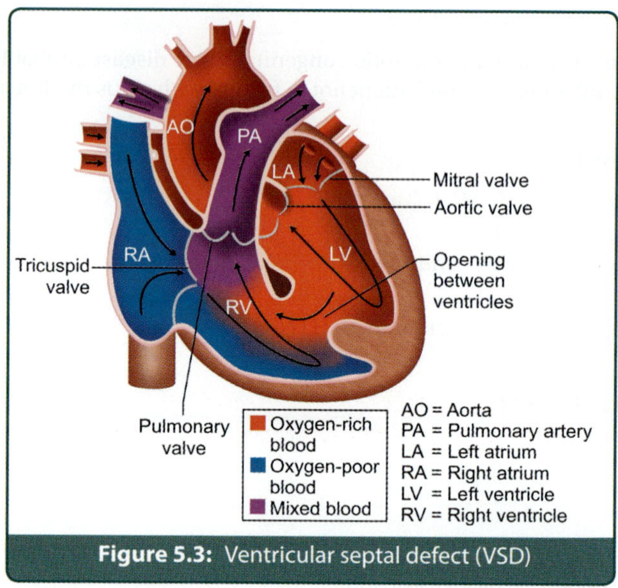

Figure 5.3: Ventricular septal defect (VSD)

Elfin facies: Supravalvular stenosis or pulmonary artery stenosis
- Wide mouth
- Large lips
- Widely-spaced teeth
- Broad forehead
- Pointed chin
- Protruding ear
- Eyes wide apart

CVS System Examination

- Pansystolic murmur at left 3/4 ICS
- Ejection systolic murmur at pulmonary area
- Mid-diastolic murmur at mitral area
- Wide variable S_2 (early A_2 and late P_2)
- Loud S_1.

Inspection

- Epigastric pulsation
- Precordial bulge
- Pulsation at pulmonary area

} Features of right ventricular hypertrophy

Shifted apical impulse outwards right ventricular hypertrophy.

Palpation

(Up to 4–5 years, apical impulse 4th ICS/lateral to mid-clavicular line)
- Hyperdynamic
- Parasternal heave

- Palpable P_2 (Eisenmenger develops)
- Palpable thrill (PSM).

Percussion

Note for any cardiomegaly.

Auscultation

- Pansystolic murmur (conducted) increased intensity in MA/AA/TA
- PSM (Grade 5–6) in 3rd or 4th ICS lower left sternal border with maximum intensity

Diagnosis

Congenital acyanotic heart disease, probably VSD with left to right shunt with no signs of CCF and pulmonary hypertension patient in sinus rhythm with marasmus/ kwashiorkor.

Classification

Depending on the Location

Older classification	*Newer classification*
Supracristal: Lie below pulmonary valve Infracristal: Behind the septal cup of tricuspid valve	**Perimembranous:** • Supracristal • Infracristal • Below aortic valve
	Muscular: • Inlet • Outlet (infundibular) • Trabecular: 3 types
	Trabecular: • Central muscular • Marginal muscular • Apical muscular

Depending on the Size (Fig. 5.4)

Features	*Small (restrictive VSD)*	*Moderate*	*Large*
History	• Asymptomatic • May have recurrent RTI • Diagnosed by physician	• Symptomatic • Recurrent RIT • Dyspnea in infancy • Subcostal retraction	• CCF signs at time of birth or neonatal period
Clinical findings	S_1S_2- normal Loud harsh PSM (grade 5–6) no PHT	S_1S_2 - normal PSM: Grade (3, 4) apical impulse shifted (RVH)	S_1S_2 normal grade 1, 3 PSM Congestive liver Breathlessness

Contd...

Contd...

Features	*Small (restrictive VSD)*	*Moderate*	*Large*
Funtional murmurs (increased flow through pulmonary artery with increased return to left atrium through pulmonary veins)	• No MDM in mitral area • No CCF	• MDM + in MA • PHT develops	• MDM + in mitral area • CCF develops
X- ray	Heart size normal mild cardiomegaly	Moderate	Gross cardiomegaly
ECG	LVH features	Biventricular HT (Katz-Wathtel phenomenon)	RVH predominates
Echocardiography	< 5 mm	6–10 mm	>10 mm

VSD Murmur

Look for pneumonic: PQRST

- P: Pitch (high pitch)
- Q: Quality (harsh)
- R: Radiates to subxiphoid
- S: Site—sternum left side
- T: Thrill

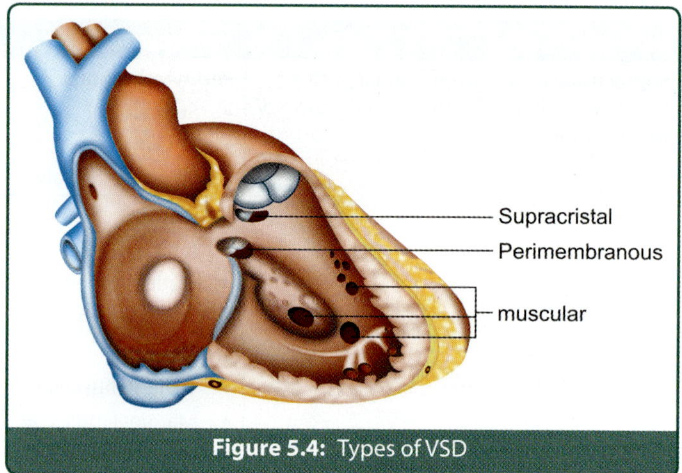

Figure 5.4: Types of VSD

Large VSD With Reversal

H/O: Cyanosis
Respiratory distress

Clinical Features

- Cyanosis
  - Clubbing +
  - S_1S_2: well heard
  - P_2 may be single/loud
  - PSM (3-5/6) grade

VSD with reversal: Eisenmengers complex—Pulmonary hypertension with VSD having Right to left shunt

Eisenmenger's complex: Development of reversal of shunt due to pulmonary hypertension

ECG: Right ventricular hypertrophy
X-ray: Hilar Pulmonary artery enlarges and peripheral lung fields becomes oligemic

Katz Wachtel Phenomenon

Equiphasic R, S waves in leads V_2, V_3, V_4 showing biventricular hypertrophy.

Maladie de Roger Syndrome

- Small VSD produces grade 5/6 PSM thrill
- Large VSD produces PSM of low intensity

Name the conditions where you get precordial bulge?

- Right ventricular hypertrophy
- Left atrial hypertrophy

Restrictive VSD: Offers high degree of rectrictive at the septum.

Nonrestrictive VSD: No resistance at the septum, but present at pulmonary circulation.

Management

Investigations

1. **Blood:** TC/DC/RBC count, Hb%, PCV
2. **Urine:** albumin (R/O hypoalbuminemia as the child may have renal problem which may be cause for her edema
3. **X-ray chest:** Cardiomegaly
4. **Serum electrolytes:** CCF to be treated with digoxin (Potassium levels to be monitored to give digoxin)
5. Blood urea
6. **ECG:** LVH/RVH features (Fig. 5.5)
   - ECG pattern depends on size of VSD
   - Large VSD will have biventricular hypertrophy: Equiphasic tall R and S waves in V_1–V_3
7. Echocardigraphy

Treatment

Medical Management

General measures

1. Maintain good dental hygiene, give prophylaxis against infective endocarditis
2. Treatment of CCF: Digoxin/diuretics/ACE inhibitors
3. Treatment of recurrent RTI
4. High calorie intake, correct anemia (since it may worsen CCF)

Spontaneous closure of VSD

- Proliferation of fibrous tissue
- Tricuspid valve closing the defect
- Aneurysm of aorta over riding the defect

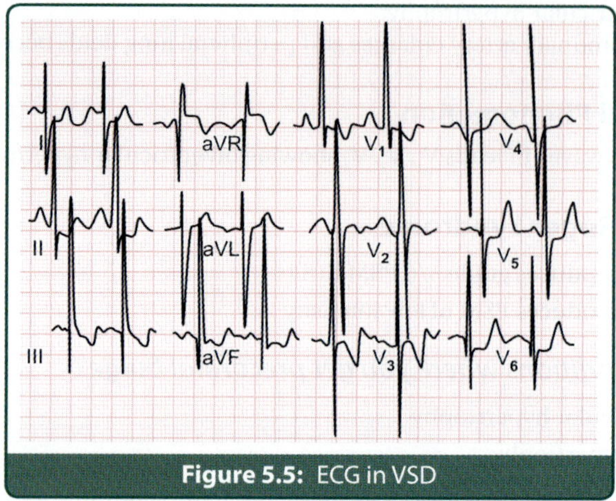

Figure 5.5: ECG in VSD

- Pseudoaneurysm
  - 30% spontaneous closure by 1 year
  - 50% spontaneous closure by 3 years
  - 80% spontaneous closure by 5 years
    Muscular type closes earlier.

Surgical Treatment

- Using a patch of woven Dacron or PTFE as it obviates
- Approach through right atrium or right ventriculotomy.

Indications

- Not closes by 5 years
- CCF not responding to medical treatment
- QP (Pulmonary Blood flow)
  QS (Systemic Blood flow)
  QP:QS > 2:1 ratio
- Rapidly rising PHT
- Even one episode of IE
- Parental anxiety

Contraindications

- Small VSD, no CHF
- QP:QS < 1.5:1
- Predominant R → L shunt
- Established PHT

Juxtaarterial VSD: (AR + VSD)

- **Absolute indication** in cause where AR (Aortic incompetence) has developed
- Approach: Transpulmonary
  Transatrial and transpulmonary (combination)

Sieve-like pores type VSD: Poor prognosis
Palliative pulmonary artery banding:
To decrease R → L shunting

Complications of VSD surgery:
- Complete heart block
- Bifascicular block
- Residual or reopened VSD.

Established pulmonary hypertension or Eisenmenger's complex the treatment option is only heart lung transplantation

TETRALOGY OF FALLOT

History Related to TOF

- H/O Cyanotic spells
- H/O Neurological deficit (convulsion, hemiplegia)
- H/O Dyspnea on exertion
- H/O Bleeding manifests
- H/O Headache, gout, polycythemia
- H/O Fever (infective endocarditis, brain abscess).

Etiology

- Commonest congenital heart disease above 2 years of age (25% of cyanotics)
- 80–100 for 10,000 population i.e., 8–10/1,000 population

Components of TOF (Fig. 5.6)

1. Infundibular stenosis of PA (RV outflow obstruction)
2. Large nonrestrictive type of VSD
3. Right ventricular hypertrophy
4. Over-riding aorta (Biventricular origin of aorta)

Right outflow through ventricle i.e., pulmonary artery; may be
  i. Infundibular stenosis (80%)
  ii. Valvular (20%).

Embryology

Truncus arteriosus gives two parts: Aorta and pulmonary artery.

The truncus arteriosus has a septum to divide the aorta/PA-conotruncal/infundibular septum → spiral septum which divides the pulmonary artery and aorta.

In tetralogy of Fallot, spiral septum is displaced anterior and cephalad direction→small pulmonary artery, over riding aorta.

Embroyological anomaly: Antero-cephalad malalignment of infundibular septum.

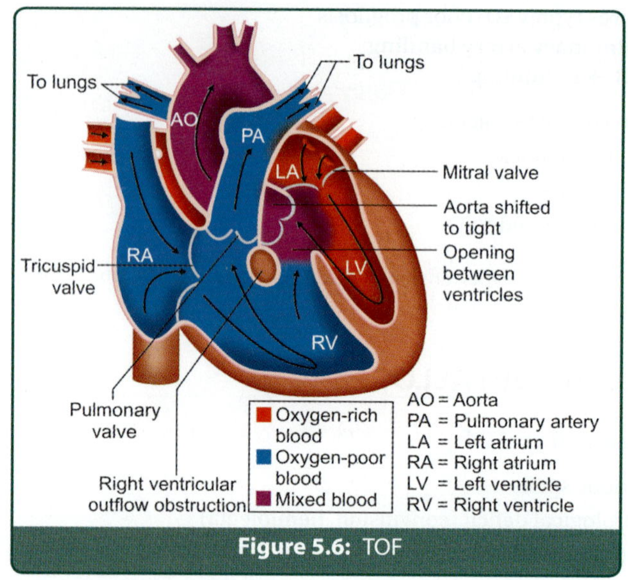

Figure 5.6: TOF

Associated Anomalies in TOF

1. Right side aortic arch (25%)
2. Left side superior vena cava
3. Associated: ASD, PDA, coarctation of aorta
4. Anomalous origin of left coronary artery
5. Dextrocardia
6. Berry aneurysm.

Syndromes Associated with TOF

1. Poland's syndrome: TOF + absent pectoral mayor (left)
2. Goldenha'r syndrome: TOF + oculoauriculovertebral dysplasia
3. Digeorge syndrome: TOF + immunodeficiency
4. Klippel-Feil syndrome: TOF + fused cervical vertebra
5. Laurence-Moon-Biedl: TOF + hypogonadism + retinitis pigmentosa + polydactyly + obesity
6. Fetal alcohol syndrome
7. CHARGE association:
   - C: Coloboma
   - H: Heart anomaly (TOF/VSD)
   - A: Choanal atresia
   - R: Renal anomaly
   - G: Growth retardation
   - E: Ear anomaly
8. TAR syndrome: Thrombocytopenia + Absent/hypoplastic radii + TOF/VSD
9. Down's syndrome: TOF + VSD + ASD

Fallot's triology: ASD + PS + Right ventricular hypertrophy (no VSD)
Fallot's pentology: ASD + TOF.

Hemodynamics (Flow Chart 5.1)

- Severity is directly proportional to cyanosis and inversely proportional to the intensity of systolic murmur (severity of pulmonary stenosis)

Right ventricular outflow obstruction: Delayed P_2

- P_2 is also reduced in intensity (not audible)
- S_2 is, therefore, single and loud A_2 (as the aortic valve is anteriorly displaced)
- Ejection click at aorta
- Because of RVH: Decreased blood flow from right atrium, hence, will have large *a'* waves in JVP.

Compensatory Mechanisms in TOF

To increase blood flow to lungs:

a. Systemic arterial collaterals: Bronchial collaterals and direct collaterals from descending aorta
b. Fistula between pulmonary and coronary arteries
c. Patent ductus arteriosus (PDA).

Pathophysiology of Cyanosis

Infundibular stenosis + large VSD + over-riding aorta

↓

More amount of deoxygenated blood enters aorta resulting in cyanosis

Flow chart 5.1: TOF

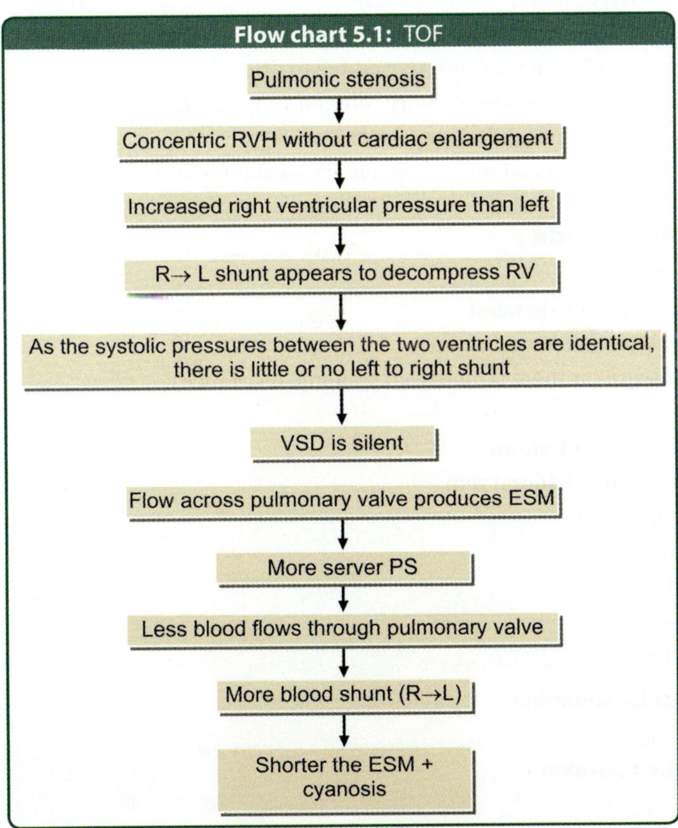

Cyanotic Spells

Why in TOF Cyanosis Occurs > 6 Months of Life?

Remember adult hemoglobin is responsible for cyanosis

i. ↑O_2 binding capacity of fetal Hb
ii. Hb fetal type is present upto 6 months
iii. Reduced pulmonary vascular resistance in neonate and more shunt left to right
iv. O_2 requirement (demand) is less in infants
v. Neonatal baby dose not cry more and lies silent whereas infants cry more resulting in cyanosis
vi. Sensitivity of infundibular receptors for catecholamines not well-developed

Cyanotic (Hypoxic) Spells

It is a vicious cycle with paroxysmal spell occurs when the baby cries in early morning hours associated with:

- Deepening of cyanosis
- Decreasing intensity of ejection systolic murmur
- Hyper (tachypnea)
- May develop fits at times

Treatment of Cyanotic Spells

i. Knee chest position
ii. Humidified O_2 therapy: ↑O_2 content
iii. Acidosis : To prevent stimulation of respiratory center
    Na bicarbonate: 2–3 meq/kg added to drip
iv. Morphine: Depresses respiratory center 0.1 mg/kg SC
v. Propranolol: ↓ infundibular spasm 0.1 mg/kg slow IV
vi. Phenylephrine injection: To ↑systemic vascular resistance

Squatting Episode

Mechanism:

1. Rest decreases O_2 demand
2. Compression of femoral artery:
   ↑LV pressure (as there is increased systemic resistance)
   ↓
   Decrease of R → L shunt
3. Compression of femoral vein:
   ↓Venous return
   ↓
   ↓R → L shunt
   ↓
   ↓Cyanosis

Equivalents for squatting:

1. Squatting
2. Knee chest position

3. Knee abdomen position
4. Scissoring the lower limb
5. Sitting with arms drawn underneath
6. Standing on one leg
7. Mother holding infant with thighs flexed
8. Lying supine
9. In infants: Put the child over the mother's shoulder.

Clinical Features

General Examination

- Cyanosis
- Tachypnea
- Clubbing
- JVP: *a*′ wave prominent
- Polycythemia (conjunctival suffusion)
- Growth retardation
- Failure to thrive

CCF will Never Occur in TOF

That is non-restrictive VSD ← no volume overload, all blood is diverted to aorta

If occurs R/O

- Anemia
- Hypertension
- Infective endocarditis
- Myocarditis
- Other valve anomalies

Palpation: Systolic thrill in pulmonary area (<30%)

Auscultation:

- S_1 normal
- S_2 single loud A_2
- ESM in pulmonary area
- Constant ejection click: Large aorta
- Inconstant ejection click: Valvular PS
- Bilateral symmetrical systolic murmur in infraclavicular/clavicular/supraclavicular —bronchopulmonary collaterals.

Investigations

1. **Blood:** TC/DC
   - Hb% → In TOF: Because of polycythemia we, cannot detect anemia
   - PCV: Most reliable to find anemia
     Keep PCV <60%
     If PCV ↑ >65%—start treatment

2. **X-ray chest:**
   - "Coeur en sabot, boot-shaped heart (Fig. 5.7)
   - RVH
   - Prominent aortic arch
     'The side of arch is indicated by the presence of concave depression of the arch on the tracheal shadow'
   - Pulmonary oligemic fields
   - Notching of ribs → stretching of vessels (increased collaterals in right).
3. **ECG**: RAD (+120 degrees to +150 degrees) in cyanotic form (Fig. 5.8)
   Tall R wave in V_1 abruptly changes to an rS in V_2.
4. **Echo**: Demonstrate all defects
   Posterior great vessel being aorta.

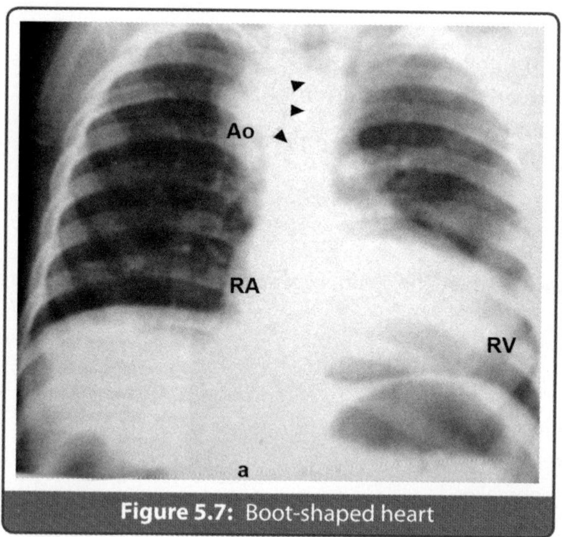

Figure 5.7: Boot-shaped heart

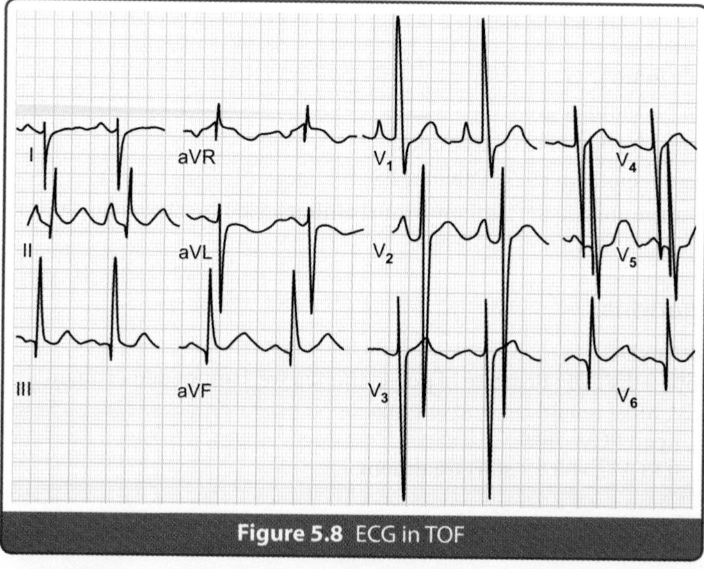

Figure 5.8 ECG in TOF

Complications (Fig. 5.2)

1. Cyanotic spells
2. Growth retardation: Most energy is used for squatting/cyanotic spells
3. Mental retardation
4. Headache from childhood due to polycythemia
5. Child > 2 years: Cerebral abscess
   Portal of entry through teeth and gums, through caries teeth enters circulation (mechanism not known)
6. **Cerebral thromboembolism** in those < 2 years, because dehydration with diarrhea is a frequent feature for less than 2 years
   ↓
   Hypovolemia + polycythemia
   ↓
   Thombus
7. **Hemiplegia:** Because of cerebral infarct (Thromboembolic manifest)
8. **Iron deficiency anemia:** Increased RBC production overtakes iron stores
9. **Tuberculous:** Due to pulmonary oligemia
10. **Infective endocarditis** (do not commit it is doubtful and contradiction)
11. **Fits:** Due to cerebral abscess/↑ ICT.

Medical Management

1. Treatment of cyanotic spells
2. Treatment of anemia (iron folic acid tablets): Depending on PCV value
3. Infective endocarditis is not common
4. Long-term propranolol
   To decrease cyanosis: 1mg/kg as a single dose
   - Decrease spasm
   - Decreases heart rate
   - Decreases cardiac output
5. If PCV >65% (Polycythemia) → Exchange transfusion with normal saline.

Surgical Management

Flow chart 5.2: Complications of polycythemia

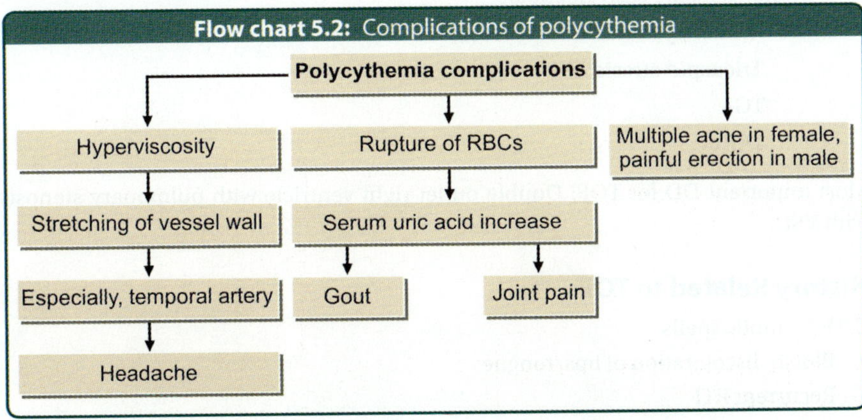

Palliative

1. **Blalock-Taussig shunt**: (>3 months age) Line, on the side opposite to aortic arch R/L subclavian artery with R/L pulmonary artery.
2. **Modified Blalock Taussig**: (< 3 months of age) 'Goretex interposition shunt' Placed between subclavian artery and ipsilateral artery.
3. **Potts shunt**: Descending aorta to left pulmonary artery.
4. **Waterston shunt**: Ascending aorta to right pulmonary A.
5. **Davidsons operation**: Ascending aorta to pulmonary trunk anastomosis.
6. **Glens operation**: (for tricuspid atresia) SVC with pulmonary artery anastomosis.

Definite

Ideal age: 3–5 years

Brock's Procedure

- Closing VSD
- Resecting infundibular obstruction.

Complications

1. Right bundle branch block (RBBB) with or without left anterior hemiblock
2. Complete heart block
3. Residual VSD/PS
4. Pulmonary regurgitation

Definite Procedure

Complete correction of TOF = Lilley's procedure.

Important points to remember in TOF

1. No VSD murmur/on ESM at PS
2. Loud ESM: Good prognosis
3. Importance of respiratory system examination: Continuous murmur

   Central nervous system examination: Plantar extensor + (cerebral thrombus/abscess)
4. If cyanotic occurs early neonatal
   - R/O either cyanotic heart diseases

     Tricuspid atresia ASD

     TGA

     TAPVC

Most important DD for TOF: Double outlet right ventricle with pulmonary stenosis with VSD.

History Related to TOF

C/O: Cyanotic spells

- Bluish discoloration of lips/tongue
- Recurrent RTI

History of Presenting Illness

- H/O Fever: IE/cerebral abscess
- H/O CNS: Convulsions/hemiplegia
- H/O Growth retardation
- H/O Headache: Polycythemia
- H/O TB
- H/O Blooding manifests
- H/O Joint pains: Polycythemia → Gout
- Recent H/O Diarrhea/vomiting: Hemoconcentration → stasis → thrombus
- H/O Loss of weight/FTT

Antenatal History

- Diabetes mellitus: Cardiomyopathy, TGA, IV septum—asymmetrical HT
- Phenytoin: TOF
- OCP: TGA
- Lithium: Ebstein's anomaly + tricuspid atresia
- Rubella: Pulmonary artery stenosis + VSD + TDA
- Mumps: Endocardial fibroelastosis

ATRIAL SEPTAL DEFECT (FIGS 5.9 AND 5.10)

Hemodynamics

- Pulmonary valve closes late: P_2 delayed
  RV fully loaded, so no increase in volume during inspiration: wide-fixed split
- P_2 accentuated
- Lung fields plethoric due to increase in blood

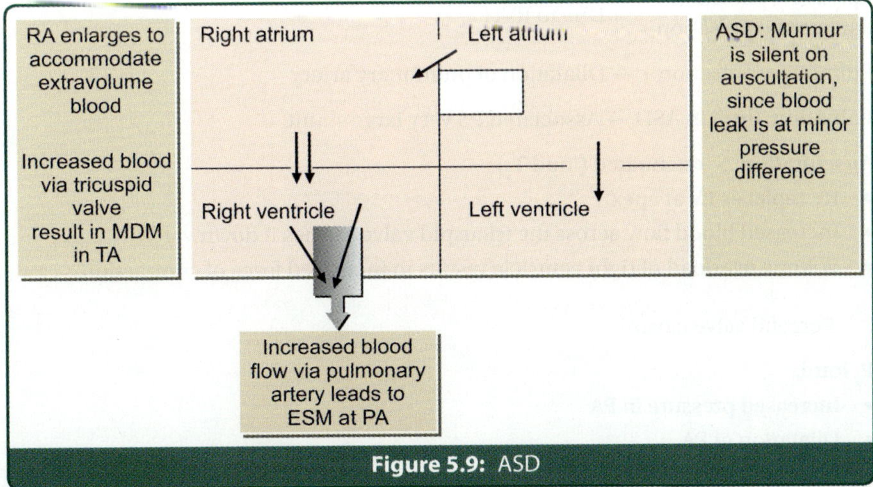

Figure 5.9: ASD

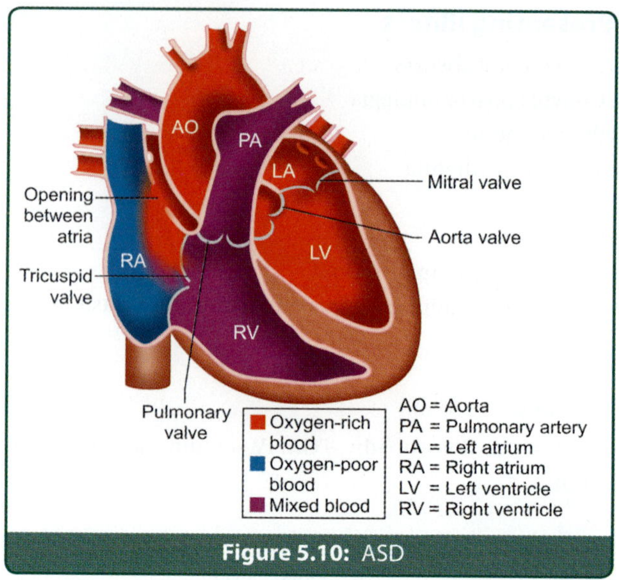

Figure 5.10: ASD

Clinical Picture

Symptoms: Asymptomatic

- Mild effort intolerance
- Frequent chest infections

G/E: No cyanosis/no clubbing
Signs: BP: N/low systolic
Pulse: N/low volume
JVP: ↑

Inspection:
Epigastric pulsation +
Parasternal pulsation + } Due to RVH

Pulmonary pulsation + → Dilatation of pulmonary artery

Palpation: thrill in ASD → Associated PS very large shunt

Auscultation: S_1 attenuated (loud T_1)

- RV replaces LV at apex
- Increased blood flow across the tricuspid valve pushes it downwards
- Volume overload of right ventricle results in increased force of contraction
  ↓
  Forceful valve closure

P_2 loud:

- Increased pressure in PA
- Dilatation of PA
- Wide split fixed

Why there is a click in ASD?

1. Pulmonary vascular click: Due to PA dilatation
2. Valvular click due to pulmonary stenosis
3. MVPS

Murmurs

- MDM at tricuspid valve
- ESM at pulmonary valve
- EDM at pulmonary area due to PR

  Causes for pansystolic murmur at mitral area:
  1. Ostium primum ASD: ECG shows left axis deviation more than 30 degrees
  2. Floppy mitral valve: (MVPS)
     (have a midsystolic click ,late ESM/PSM)
  3. Ostium secundum + rheumatic MR
  4. Ostium secundum + cleft mitral valve (Rare)

  } Right axis deviation
- Severity of ASD is shown by intensity of murmur and heart size

Complications

1. Recurrent respiratory tract infection
2. Pulmonary HT → Disappearance of murmurs with ejection click and palpable P_2; But S_2 widely split
3. Paradoxical emboli
4. Atrial fibrillation
5. CCF
6. Infective endocarditis (very rare)

Investigations

X-ray Chest

- Jug handle appearance (Dilated pulmonary A)
- Mild to moderate cardiomegaly
- RA, RV enlargement
- Prominent main PA segment
- Relatively small aortic shadow
- Plethoric lung fields

ECG (5.11)

- Ostium secundum: Right axis deviation; RVH
- Ostium primum: Lt axis deviation beyond 30
- RBBB with rsR\` V_1

ECHO: ↑RV size
Paradoxical ventricular septal motion.

In older children → transesophageal echocardiography needed to visualize the defect.

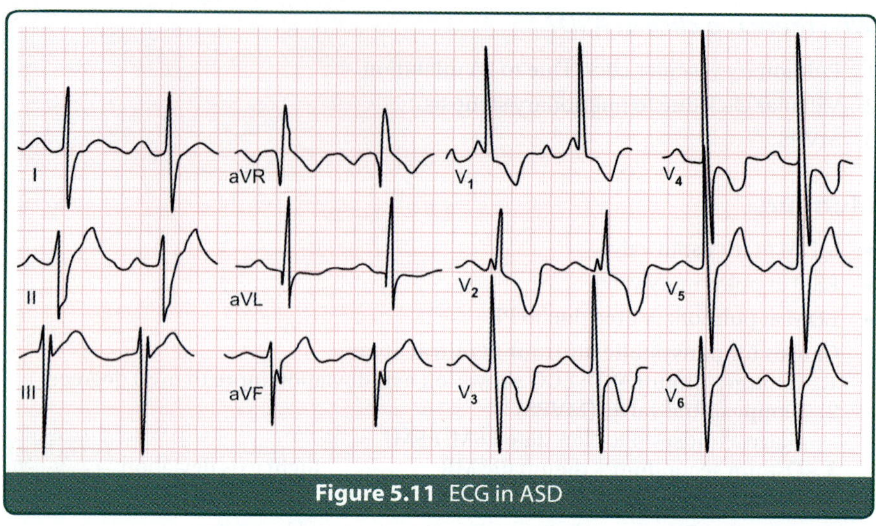

Figure 5.11 ECG in ASD

Treatment

Medical

i. No exercise restriction
ii. Treat CHF in infants
iii. For chest infection
iv. Non-surgical closure indicated nowadays by 'Clamshell' or 'buttoned' devices in uncomplicated smaller devices.

Surgical

- Natural H/O: <3 mm—spontaneous closure in 100% by 1 and half years
- Infective endocarditis do not occurs (no need of prophylaxis)
- >8 mm: Rarely closes spontaneously.

Indications of Surgery

1. Left to right shunt with QP/QS >1.5.
2. Some consider small ASD → because of risk of paradoxical emboli and CVA.

Contraindication

- PVR: >10 units/m^2 (Normal: 1–3 units)
- Ideal age: 2–4 years (spontaneous closure <2years)
- But if CHF does not responds to medical treatment, do surgery
- Closed by suturing or pericardial or a teflon patch or prolene mesh.

Complications

Immediate postoperative: Arrhythmia, CVA
<1%: Death
Sick sinus syndrome: In repair of sinus venous defect

Types of ASD (Fig. 5.12)

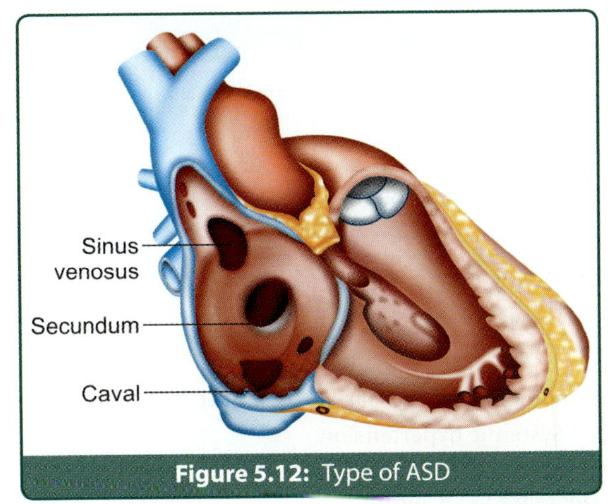

Figure 5.12: Type of ASD

1. **Ostium secundum (commonest) 50–70%:** located at fossa ovalis associated MPS
2. **Ostium primum defect (3%):** Common in Down's syndrome associated with cleft anterior mitral leaflet, with or without cleft in septal tricuspid leaflet.
3. **Sinus venosus ASD (10%) at the level of**
   i. **SVC**: Usually associated
      1. Biatrial connectional SVC
      2. TAPVC

   ii. **IVC**

   iii. **Coronary sinus.**

Syndromes Associated with ASD

1. Down's syndrome: Ostium primum ASD
2. Holt Oram syndrome: (familial) triphalangism of thumb hypoplasia of 1st MC bone. Absent radius and ASD
3. Ellis-van Creveld syndrome:
   - ASD with polydactylism (post axial)
   - Multiple frenula connecting upper lip with gums
   - Neonatal teeth
   - Single atrium
4. Patau (Trisomy:13)
5. Edward (Trisomy:18)
6. Lutembacher (ASD + acquired MS)
7. Noonan syndrome (mainly PS/ASD)

Differential Diagnosis

1. Rheumatic MS
2. PS
3. Supracrystal VSD
4. PHT
5. Idiopathic dilatation of PA
6. Straight back syndrome (pectus excavatum)

Ostium primum	*Ostium secundum*
10–15% of ASD	80–85% of ASD
Male = Female	Female > male
Associated with MR/TR	Associated with MVPS
Increased L → R shunt	Mild
PHT: early	Late
Poor prognosis	Good
ECG-LAD (30 degrees)	RAD (Right axis deviation)

Conditions that **Increase L→R shunt**

1. Systemic hypertension
2. AS

Decrease L→R shunt:

1. PS (pulmonary stenosis)
2. PHT

Surgery induced (Iatrogenic) ASD → while doing mitral valvotomy (CMC) (closed mitral commissurotomy)

- **To operate below 2 years:** Hypothermia induced and operated

Ideal age of correction:
ASD: 2–4 years
VSD: >5 years
PDA: <2 years

- CCF develops in
  - VSD } 1–2 months (Max 6 weeks)
  - PDA }
- CCF never develops in ASD
  - In 4–10 weeks
  - If findings suggestive of ASD with cyanosis/CCF
    ↓
    R/O: TAPVC

PATENT DUCTUS ARTERIOSUS (PDA) (FIGS 5.13 AND 5.14)

- Proximal part of left 6th aortic arch becomes proximal segment of left pulmonary artery
- Distal part of left 6th aortic arch persists as ductus arteriosus which is attached to aorta distal to left subclavian

After Birth

Functional closure after birth (24–48 hours)
Anatomical changes: 4 weeks: sclerosis (10–21 days)
↓
Converted to ligamentum arteriosum
In premature baby: 3 months

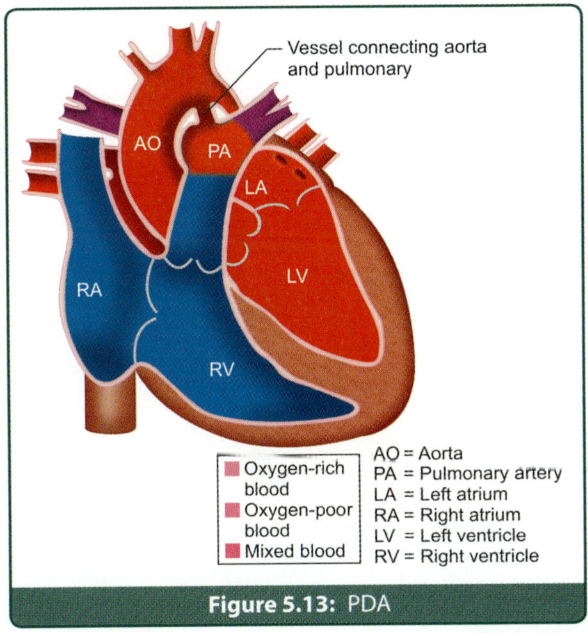

Figure 5.13: PDA

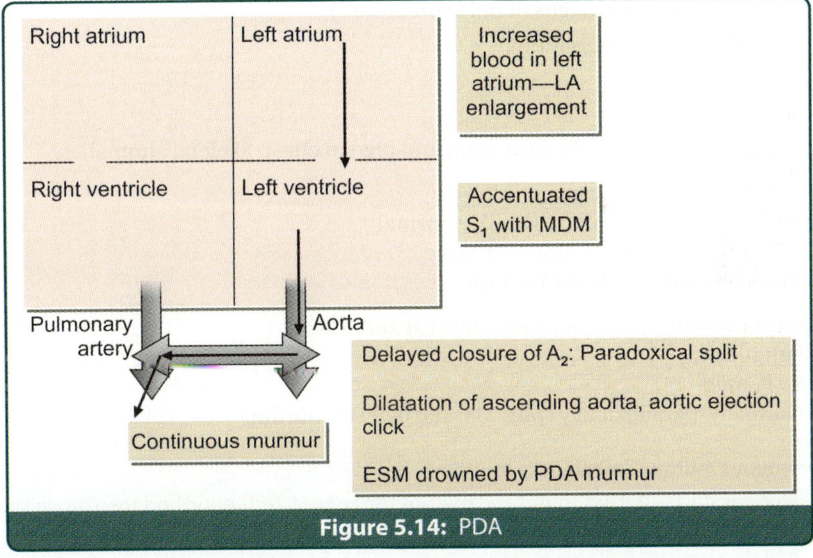

Figure 5.14: PDA

PDA: PDA is a communication between the PA and aorta
Incidence: sex ratio—F:M = 3:1
↑incidence in high altitudes
Maternal infection → in 1st trimester
↓
PDA

HEMODYNAMICS IN PDA

Syndromes associated PDA:

- Rubella syndrome
- Patau (Tri-13)
- Edward (Tri-18)

Clinical Picture

Develop CCF around 6–10 weeks of age

In older children

- Effort intolerance
- Palpitation
- Frequent chest infection.

Dilated pulmonary artery → compresses recurrent laryngeal nerve
↓
Hoarseness of voice (Ortner's syndrome)

On Examination

General Examination

- Wide pulse pressure (signs of pulse pressure↑)
- Prominent carotid pulsations +
- Collapsing pulse
- ↓Diastolic pressure
- Harrison groove, pectus excavatum and pigeon chest: Skeletal anomalies.

Pulse: Collapsing character
Inspection: Uncomplicated PDA: JVP normal
PDA with PHT → Prominent *'a'* wave
Apical impulse → Hyperdynamic

Palpation: Systolic (or) continuous thrill at 2nd ICS
Auscultation: S_1↑↑
S_2: P_2 loud
Normally/paradoxically split: Masked by PDA murmur

Continuous murmur (machinery murmur)

- Murmur starts after 1st sound and reaches the peak at 2nd sound and then diminishes in intensity and is audible only during part of diastole. (1/3rd)
- Systolic → Grating rough murmur and is broken into multiple systolic sounds. (Multiple click)
- Peak around 2nd sound: Differentiates it from other continuous murmur
- Best heard at 2nd ICS, just below left clavicle

Assessment of Severity

- Heart size
- Third heart sound → large shunt
- Delayed diastolic murmur → large shunt
- Wide pulse pressure.

Complications

- CCF
- PHT

  Features:
  - P_2 palpable
  - During diastole: Pressure in aorta and PA are equal, hence, only systolic murmur
  - As pulmonary artery pressure ↑→ ESM is heard
  - Reversal of shunt occurs
    No murmur
    Silent PDA
  - Differential cyanosis
    Toes cyanosed
    Digits not cyanosed
- Reversal → Eisenmenger's syndrome
- IE → Infective arteritis
- Dissection of ductus.

On setting of pulmonary hypertension:
- The continuous machinery murmur becomes silent, only ESM is heard; P_2 is loud at pulmonary area

Differential Diagnosis (DD)

- **For continuous murmur:**
  - Coronary A-V fistula
  - Rupture of sinus valsalva
  - Aortic pulmonary septal defect
  - Systemic A-V fistula over chest
  - Bronchial collateral murmur
  - Pulmonary A-V fistula
  - Peripheral pulmonic stenosis
  - Venous hum (TAPVC)
  - Small ASD with MS
- **Impression of continuous murmur due to PSM and diastolic**
  - VSD with AR
  - AR + MR

  AS + AR never gives an auscultatory impression of continous murmur.

Natural History

- Unlike PDA in preterm, spontaneous closure of the PDA does not occur.

Treatment

Medical

i. No exercise restriction in absence of PHT
ii. Indomethacin (is ineffective in term infant, useful only in preterm)
    Diagnosed <2 weeks age
    Indomethacin (PG synthetase inhibitor)
    0.1 mg/kg orally 12 hourly, 3 doses
    Contraindication: Hepatic/renal insufficiency

iii. SABE prophylaxis (small PDA)
iv. Experimental stage: Double umbrella device, adjustable buttoned device, by catheteral closure.

Surgical Induction

Anatomic existence of PDA, regardless of size in an indication for surgery

- Ideal age: 6 months–2 years
- Any time in old children.

Procedure

Ligation and division through left posterolateral thoracotomy without cardiopulmonary bypass.

Death <1%

When will you get mixed cyanosis?

CCF/LVF-(cyanosis both central/peripheral)

Where will you get Harrison's sulcus?

- Just above subcostal margin
- Only in infants due to pliable ribs
- Occurs in L → R shunt: Due to recurrent RTI
- It is an indication of chronic RTI

When will reversal of shunt occurs? (↑pulmonary HTN)

- PDA: 2 decade (10–20 years)
- VSD: 3rd decade (20–30 years)
- ASD: 4th decade (30–40 years)

Acute Rheumatic Fever

Definition

The RF is a postinfectious, immunologic disease that results either from:

i. Heightened immunologic reactivity to streptococcal antigens that evoke antibodies cross reactive with human tissue antisera.
(or)
ii. Some form of autoimmune reaction incited by streptococcal infection.

2002–2003, WHO, criteria for the diagnosis of rheumatic fever and rheumatic heart disease (based on the revised Jones criteria)

Diagnostic categories	*Criteria*
Primary episode of RF	Two major *or one major and two minor** manifestations plus evidence of a preceding group A streptococcal infection***
Recurrent attack of RF in a patient without established rheumatic heart disease	Two major or one major and two minor manifestations plus evidence of a preceding group A streptococcal infection
Recurrent attack of RF in a patient with established rheumatic heart disease	Two minor manifestations plus evidence of a preceding group A streptococcal infection

Contd...

Contd...

Diagnostic categories	*Criteria*
Rheumatic chorea Insidious onset rheumatic carditis	Other major manifestations or evidence of group A streptococcal infection not required
Chronic valve lesions of RHD (patients presenting for the first time with pure mitral stenosis or mixed mitral valve disease and/or aortic valve disease)	Do not require any other criteria to be diagnosed as having rheumatic heart disease

* Major manifestations	• Carditis • Polyarthritis • Chorea • Erythema marginatum • Subcutaneous nodules
** Minor manifestations	• Clinical: fever, polyarthralgia • Laboratory: elevated acute phase reactants (erythrocyte sedimentation rate or leukocyte count) • Electrocardiogram: prolonged P-R interval
*** Supporting evidence of a preceding streptococcal infection within the last 45 days	• Elevated or rising antistreptolysin-O or other streptococcal antibody, or • A positive throat culture, or • Rapid antigen test for group A streptococci, or • Recent scarlet fever

Jones Criteria

1. Either 2 major criteria
2. 1 major and 2 minor criteria
3. In pediatric cases:

   RF confirmed by

   a. Chorea (unless otherwise proved)
      (where 1 major itself is enough)
      (or)

   b. Previous H/O rheumatic fever

Incidence: 5.7/1000 (6–16 years age group)
Prevalence: 0.55/1000

Describe the pathology of pancarditis?

- **Aschoff bodies**: Foci of fibrinoid necrosis surrounded by lymphocytes, macrophages and occasional plasma cells, plump activated histocytes called aschoff cells (or) anitschkow cells.

Aschoff cells

- Amphophilic cytoplasm
- Central round to avoid nuclei
- Chromatin is dispersed in a central, slender wavy ribbon resembling cater pillar cells

  i. **Pericarditis:** Serofibrinous or serosanguinous exudates present in between pericardium and heart (bread and butter pericaritis)

  ii. **Myocarditis:** Flabby myocardium (grossly)

     Myocardial fibers separated by inflammatory cells and aschoff nodules

iii. **Endocarditis:** Verrucous small vegetations made up of fibrin, platelets and engulfed WBCs and RBCs

↓

Present in cuspal (Atrial surface) chordal, commissural

- Scarring of cuspal and commissural shortening of chorda tendinae.

Which is the commonest manifestation of rheumatic fever?

1. Polyarthritis (70–80%)
2. Carditis (50–60%)
3. Chorea (15%)
4. Subcutaneous nodules (<5%)
5. Erythema nodosum (1%)

Describe polyarthritis

- Commonest manifest of RF
- Affects large joints
- Migratory in nature
- Flitting and fleeting type with no sequelae

(Flitting—severe; Fleeting—early recover)

The arthritis dramatically responds to salicylates in 48 hours; if not responds, the diagnosis of RF is incorrect.

Describe Erythema Marginatum

- Non-itchy, erythematous
- Central clearing
- Serpiginous borders
- Rashes disappear on exposure to cold and reappear when covered with warm blanket
- Most prominent on trunks and inner proximal portions of extremities
- Never occurs in face

What do you mean by primary prophylaxis/secondary prophylaxis of RF?

Primary prophylaxis:

- The patient has no RF
- Then risk population with low socioeconomic group with sore throat screened for β-hemolytic *Streptococcus* by throat swab
- Primary prophylaxis is given to prevent 1st attack of RF. We give any one of the following drugs

1. Procaine penicillin: Daily IM for 10 days 4.6 lac units
2. Oral penicillin: 50,000 units/kg BW for 10 days or 250 mg QID for 10 days
3. Cephalexin: 40 mg/kg BW tds/10 days
4. Amoxicillin/ampicillin
   - Sulfonamides and tetracycline are not given
   - Erythromycin not used for primary prevention

Secondary prophylaxis:
Long course antibiotics in a known case of/RHD/RF to prevent recurrence of RF

- No carditis: 5 years/18 years of age whichever is longer
- Mild: Moderate carditis—10 years/25 years of age whichever is longer
- Severe disease/postoperative RHD: Life long

Benzathine Penicillin

- <27 kg: 6,00,000 U in every 21 days
- >27 kg: 1.2 MU/IM every 21 days

Oral Penicillin

250 mg tablet: BD (each tab = 4 lac units of penicillin)

Sulfonamides

- Oral sulfadiazine: 0.5 g once a day (<27 kg)
- 1 gm a day (>27kg)

Erythromycin

40 mg/kg/24 hours orally

- For patents allergic to penicillin
- Give sulfonamides (or) erythromycin

Investigations in a Case of RF

1. Blood:
   TC leukocytosis (10,000 to 15,000/cubic mm)
   DC
   ESR ½ hour: >15 mm
   1 hour >30 mm
   affected by anemia (increased ESR) and CCF (decreased ESR)
   CRP: >20 μg/mL
2. ASO titer:
   Basal ASO titer of any individual: 50 units
   In adult, goes upto 250 units = Streptococcal infection
   Children: >330 Todd units
3. X-ray: Cardiomegaly
4. Echo: pericardial effusion
5. ECG: PR Interval↑
   Tachycardia

Treatment

1. Bed rest:
   a. Arthritis only:
      Complete bed rest: 2 weeks
      Limitation of only indoor activities: 2 weeks
      Limitation of outdoor activities: After another 4–6 weeks

b. Carditis:
   No CCF: Complete bed rest: 4 weeks
   For indoor : 4 weeks
   For outdoor: 8–10 weeks
   CCF: Complete bed rest: 3 months/till fully recovering
   Limit indoor: 4–6 weeks
   Limit outdoor: For 5 months

2. Treatment of RF:
   1. Procaine penicillin: 4–6 lac unit OD IM 10 days
   2. Penicillin G: 50,000 units/kg—every 6 hours for 10 days IV
      Allergic to penicillin—erythromycin: 40 mg/kg, QID.
   3. Anti-inflammatory treatment:
      1. Acetylsalicylic acid (aspirin):
         90–120 mg/kg 3 doses
         80–100 mg/kg 4–5 doses
      2. Steroids: 2 mg/kg per day in 4 divided doses (prednisone)

Treatment Schedule

- **Arthritis with mild carditis**: Aspirin 4 weeks + antacid only arthritis
  Mild carditis → Prednisolone for 6 weeks slowly taper
- **Moderate carditis without CCF** :
  Steroids: Prednisolone for 2 weeks (2 mg/kg in 4 divided doses) then taper for 6 weeks
  Add aspirin while tapering.
- **Carditis with CCF:**
  Steroids as above with added treatment for CCF:
  - Digoxin—half the dose
  - Furosemide
  - Fluid restriction
  - Bedrest with back rest
  - Dilators.
- **Chorea:**
  - Haloperidol: 0.5–2 mg every 8 hours
  - Phenobarbitone: 15–30 mg every 8 hours (drug of choice)
  - Chlorpromazine
  - Diazepam can be used.

CASE 6 Respiratory System

- Bronchiectasis
- Asthma
- Bronchitis
- Pleural Effusion
- Bronchopneumonia

Case: Discussion (usually RS case is not kept in exam for UG)
'Bronchopneumonia'

HISTORY

H/O Cough

- H/O Difficulty in feeding
- H/O Refusal to feed
- H/O Incessant cry
- H/O Fever
- H/O Respiratory distress

Difference:

i. Lobar pneumonia: Inflammation of lung parenchyma.
ii. Bronchopneumonia: Inflammation of periphery of bronchus/alveoli with patchy involvement of both lobes.

CLASSIFICATION

1. Viral: RSV adenosines, influenza, metapneumovirus
2. Bacterial: Staphylococcal, streptococcal, *H influenza*
3. Atypical: *Chlamydia, Mycoplasma*
4. Fungi: Histoplasmosis, coccidiomycosis
5. Helminthes: *Ascaris* (Löeffler's syndrome)
6. Aspiration: Food, oily drops
7. Hydrocarbon: Chemical pneumonitis (kerosene)
8. Lipoidal: Interstitial pneumonitis
9. Hypersensitivity

NEWBORN

Common:

1. Group B: *Streptococcus*
2. *E coli, Klebsiella*

Organisms that are present in genital tract

If a newborn baby immediately after birth presents with respiratory distress
C/O: Tachypnea

- Cyanosis
- Feeding difficulty

O/E: Fine crepts/ rhonchi

What are the 3 things to be R/O:

1. Early onset B pneumonia (Group B)
2. Septicemia
3. Meconium aspiration syndrome (commonest)

In a preterm infant with above features, we suspect:

- Hyaline membrane disease
- Early onset pneumonia

Why is it Gram-negative organisms are common but not Gram-positive in newborn?

i. IgG antibodies cross the placenta and protects against Gram-positive organisms
ii. IgM which action Gram-negative develops later.

Investigations

1. Chest X-ray
2. TC, DC
3. Gastric aspirate: Less than 5 Neutrophils = Early onset pneumonia
4. Blood culture

Treatment

- Penicillin G: 50,000 IU kg/ BW 3–5 days
- Gentamicin: 3–5 mg/kg BW 3–5 days.

FIRST 6 MONTHS

Bronchiolitis

- Respiratory syncytial virus—60%
- Adenovirus—30%, metapneumovirus

Common in winter.

- Acquired from family members
- Interferon (antiviral substance in breast milk) IgA, hence exclusively breastfed infants are not infected by RSV
- 1% mortality.

Pathophysiology

Inflammation and edema of bronchiolar mucosa

↓

Decreased ventilation

↓

Hypoxemia (↓O_2)

Hypercapnea (↑CO_2)
↓
Respiratory acidosis
↓
Hyperventilation
↓
Metabolic acidosis
↓
Respiratory failure

C/O: Acute onset

- Rhinorrhea
- Sudden onest of distress/feeding difficult
- Incessant cry/cyanosis

Grunting → closure of glottis during expiration
(Protective mechanism to increase functional capacity of lung)

Treatment: Supportive care

- Fluid replacement (as fluid lost in tachypnea), oxygen
- Antibiotics is questionable
- Ribavirin: 3% NaCl
- Nebulizers: 3–5 days
- Bronchodilators: β-adrenergic drugs, salbutamol, ipratropium (rarely needed)
- Sedation must not be given as the baby may go for respiratory depression.

Lipoidal Pneumonia (Interstitial Pneumonitis)

- H/O instilling oil in the nose (Bad home practice)
- No H/O fever
- Only cough/feeding difficulty
- Not responds to antibiotics
- Peak 6 months—4 year age
- Acute onset
- Rhinorrhea
- Sudden onset of distress/feeding/incessant cry and cyanosis

O/E: Interstitial pneumonia
Diagnosed by: Acute onset, no crepts, cyanosis +

STAPHYLOCOCCAL PNEUMONIA

Follows any skin infection (impetigo)/pyoderma that later spreads to systemic circulation.

O/E:

- Highly toxic
- Intercostal/chest retraction (Fig. 6.1)
- Grunting
- Absent breath sounds
- Septicemia

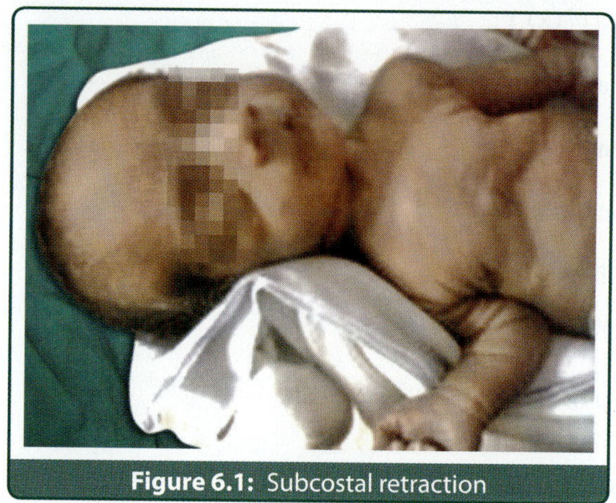

Figure 6.1: Subcostal retraction

X-ray:
- Opacity of lung
- Pneumatocele

Complication

Pneumatoceles may rupture and produce pyopneumothorax and tension pneumothorax

Rx: Intercostal drainage for empyema, pyopneumothorax
- Supportive
- Cloxacillin
- Vancomycin (for (MRSA) methicillin resistant *Staphylococcus aureus*).

HYDROCARBON PNEUMONIA

Kerosene → mainly excretion through lungs = chemical pneumonia
Common in summer → child drinks to satisfy thirst accidentally thinking as water

May also lead to:
i. Aspiration pneumonitis
ii. Secondary pneumonitis

<6 months age: Severe hypoxia → hypoxic convulsions

Treatment: Gastric wash is contraindicated (lead to aspiration)
If drinks more than 10 mL = Guarded stomach wash through endoscopic tube or Ryle's tube.

C/O:
- Fever
- Respiratory distress
- Tachypnea
- Normal for first 6 hours

Contraindication: Do not use steroids
Treatment: Supportive measures

X-ray chest = Ill-defined homogenous/patchy clouding, miliary mottling
X-ray picture appears only after.... hours and may persist for 7 days.

PNEUMOCOCCAL PNEUMONIA (SCHOOL GOING CHILDREN)

Consolidation of lung

Secondary herpetic lesions around mouth seen in only 2 conditions — pneumococcal pneumonia and malaria.

Stages

- Congestion (only absent breath sounds)
- Red hepatization (infants will have fine crepts)
- Grey hepatization (infants will have fine crepts)
- Resolution (coarse crepts)

Treatment: 50,000 U/kg/day for 7 days IV/IM penicillin G

Others

Viral pneumonia: 6 months to 2 years age

- Severely ill
- Common: RSV

Post-measles pneumonia: Interstitial pneumonia

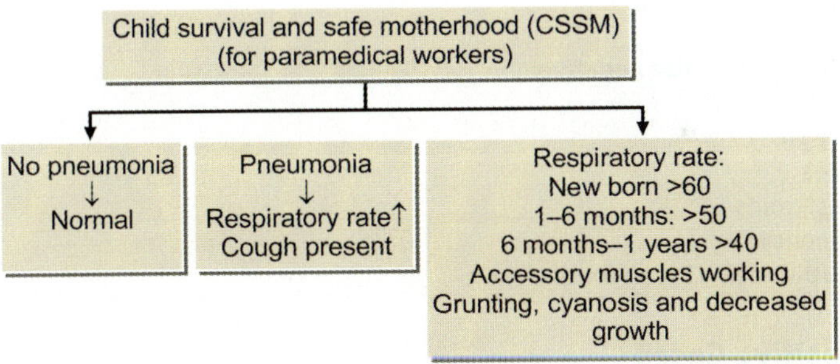

Treatment: Co-trimoxazole of tablets (IBD) for 3 days and review after 24 hours. If persists refer to hospital.

MANTOUX TEST

TEST: 0.1 mL of a suitable solution of tuberculin PPD (purified protein derivative) is injected intradermal (ID) on volar aspect of the forearm. A wheal of 5 mm should be raised.

Inference: Erythema and induration
The test result is read after 72 hours:

- <6 mm → Negative
- 6–9 mm → Doubtful
- >10 mm → Positive
- 15 mm or more → strong evidence of TB

Hyperaccelerated Mantoux—>20 mm size in 24 hours.

5 mm or more → Interpreted as positive in
i. Individuals of close contact TB
ii. X-ray reading healed TB
iii. HIV positive.

10 mm or more → Interpreted as positive in
i. High-risk groups
ii. Associated medical disease like lymphoma, malnutrition, renal failure or diabetes.

5 TU = 1 TU of PPD with RT 23 Tween 80
5 TU = 0.0001 mg PPD in 0.1 mL of diluent PPD (purified protein derivative).

Strain used for preparing is RT 23 Tween 80

BCG vaccinated cases: 4–12 weeks after immunization. Mantoux becomes positive. After 5 years it become negative.

False Negative Cases

1. Tuberulosis in incubation period or before hypersensitivity has developed
2. Following measles (for several weeks Mantoux is positive)
3. Corticosteroid treatment
4. TB meningitis or miliary TB
5. Severe malnutrition
6. Wrong technique of administration (SC)
7. Inactive tuberculin
8. Cases where CMI depressed—malignancy, Hodgkin's disease
9. Generalized anasarca.

Remember 6 M for false negative:
- Meningitis TB
- Miliary TB
- Measles
- More steroids
- Malignancy
- Malnutrition and immunodeficiency

False Positive Cases

1. After BCG vaccination
2. Leprosy, infection with other atypical mycobacteria
3. Sarcoidosis
4. Boostering effect: When a second Mantoux test after 1–2 week will become positive.

How to read Mantoux test?

- The induration is to be read horizontally and not longitudinal in the forearm.

HEAF TEST/MULTIPLE PUNCTURE TEST

Heaf gun carries a head with needle and blades. The undiluted tuberculin is injected over the skin. Heaf gun is used to pierce the tuberculin covered skin with blades. Result is read after 3–7 days.

- If there are 4 distinct papules indurated at site of injection, it is considered as positive.

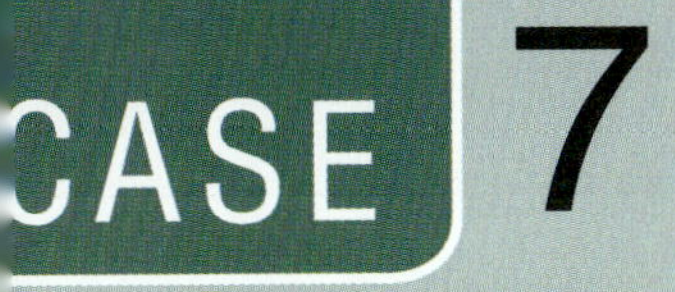

CASE 7 Newborn

CASES

Normal Newborn (Fig. 7.1)

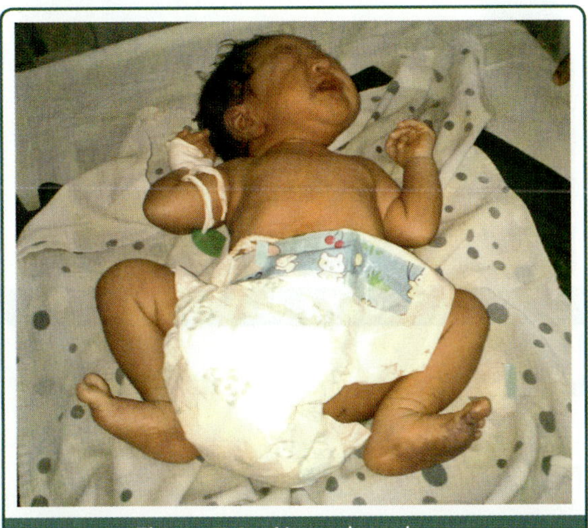

Figure 7.1: Normal newborn

Preterm (Fig. 7.2)

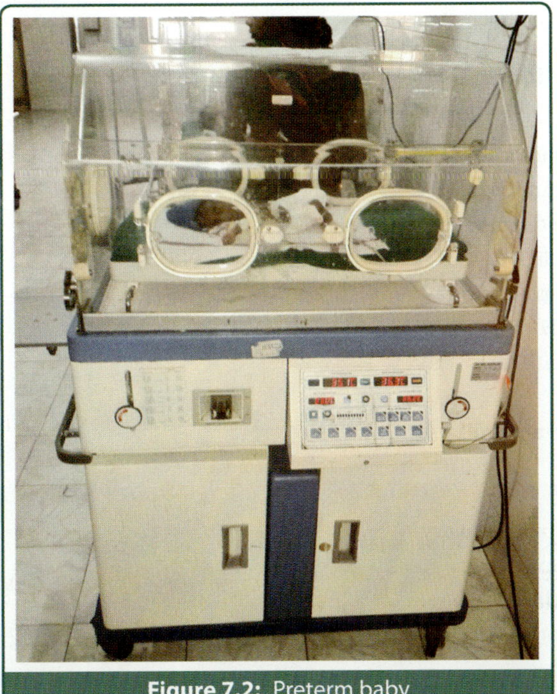

Figure 7.2: Preterm baby

IUGR (Intrauterine Growth Restriction) (Fig. 7.3)

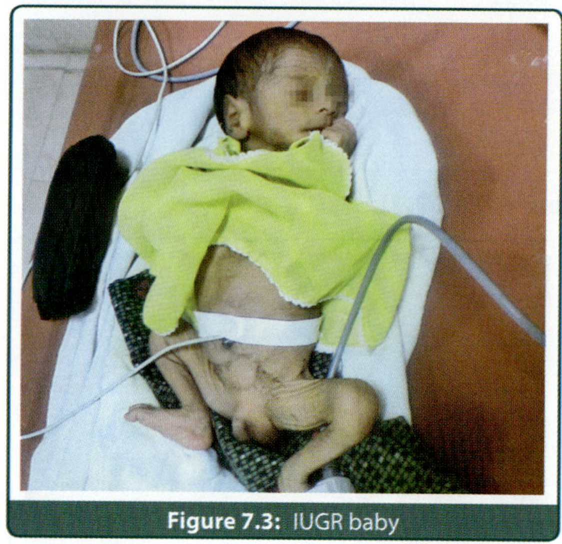

Figure 7.3: IUGR baby

Neonatal Jaundice

NEWBORN: PRETERM

History/Examination

A 20-year-old Yasodha, house wife gave birth to twins through vaginal route.

A 5-day-old female baby admitted for prematurity and LBW in neonatal ward.

Presenting complaints: Nil

Antenatal History

- Primi/multi
- No H/O previous miscarriages
- Booked/Immunized
- Iron/folic acid consumption?
- Tetanus toxoid 2 doses?
- H/O Drugs/irradiation?
- H/O DM/PIH/IHD/TB/Epilepsy
- H/O Fever with rash
- Diet
- H/O Trauma and fall.

Natal History

- Preterm hospital delivery
- Normal vertex delivery
- H/O II stage labor

- H/O Drug/transfusions
- H/O Membrane rupture (prolonged rupture of membrane (>18 hours infection)
- H/O Birth weight <1.5 kg
- H/O Child cried immediately after birth
- H/O Jaundice/color of child
- H/O Convulsions/cyanosis/respiratory distress
- APGAR score
- H/O Birth injury/deformity
- H/O Umbilical sepsis
- H/O NICU admission

Postnatal History

- H/O Breastfeeding
- Prelactic feeds
- H/O Meconium passage
- H/O Urine
- H/O Feeding difficulties

Family History

- H/O Consanguinity
- H/O Neonatal death/newborn problems

Social History

- Father's occupation } Per capita income
- Mother's occupation }
- Drinking water
- Waste disposal
- Latrine facility
- H/O Overcrowding
- Parental smoking

Immunization History

- Look for BCG scar
- OPV—0 dose given

General Examination

- Baby comfortable
- Not acutely sick
- Activity: Fair
- Cry—normal
- No paradoxical irritability
- Color: Jaundice/cyanosis
- Lanugo hair.

Normal variants in newborn:
- Erythema toxicum
- Mongolian spot
- Subconjunctival hemorrhage
- Breast enlargement
- Epstein pearl
- Natal teeth
- Vaginal bleed, discharge
- Physiological phimosis

Anthropometry

- Weight
- Height
- Weight for height
- Head circumference
- Chest circumference
- Skin fold thickness
- Quetelet index
- Ponderal index.

Head to Foot Examination

- **Head:**
  - Size
  - Shape
  - Fontanelles
  - Sutures
  - Scalp
  - Hair

Look for
- Microcephaly
- Caput, cephalhematoma
- Craniosynostosis
- Widened posterior fontanelle

- **Face:**
  - Any asymmetry
  - Bridge of nose
  - Hypertelorism
- **Eyes:**
  - Lids
  - Eyebrow and lashes
  - Conjuctiva and sclera: Hemorrhage
  - Cornea: Cataract
  - Pupils: Asymmetrical/coloboma of iris
- **Ears:**
  - Low set
  - Ear tags

  - Fistula
  - Recoiling
- **Nose:**
  - Choanal atresia
- **Mouth:**
  - Cleft lip/palate
  - Teeth
  - Tongue
- **Neck:**
  - No cysts
  - No webbed neck
  - No fistula and sinus
- **Chest:**
  - Shape/symmetry
  - Breast nodule
  - CVS: Heart rate, S1/S2
  - RS: Normal vesicular breath sounds
  - Abdomen: Shape, visible veins, distension, organomegaly, umbilical cord, hernial orifices
- **Genitalia**
  - Any vulval discharge/bleeding
  - Fusion of labia/enlargement of clitoris
  - Labium minora exposed
  - Undescended testis, scrotum rugosity, pigmentation, congenital hernia
- **Rectal**
  - Fissures
  - Fistula
  - Imperforate anus
- **Extremities**
  - No deformity
  - Digits—normal
  - Nails
  - Palmar/plantar crease
  - Arm recoil
- **Back/spine**
  - Tenderness
  - Tuft of hair
  - Mongolian spot
- **Vital Signs**
  - Pulse
  - Respiratory rate
  - Heart rate
  - Temperature.

Gestational Age Assessment

1. **New Ballard score:**

   Advantages:

   Score includes:

   1. Extreme premature infant
   2. Physical maturity
   3. Neuromuscular maturity

Physical maturity scoring ranges from –1 to +5
- Skin texture
- Lanugo
- Plantar surface
- Breast size
- Ear firmness
- Male genitals
- Female genitals.

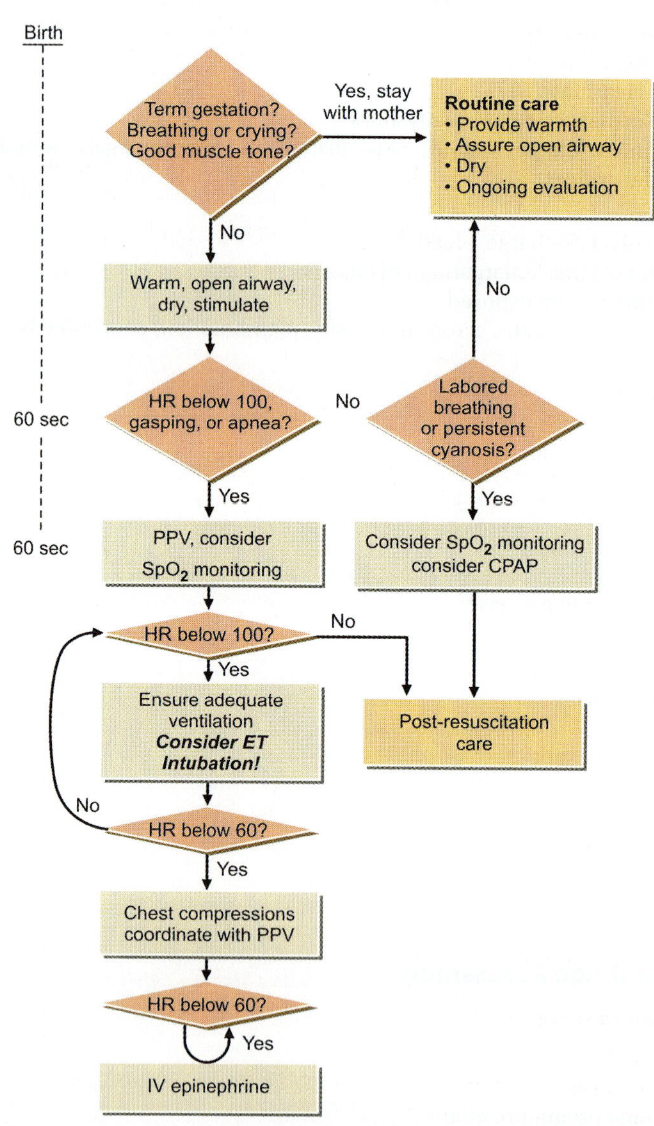

2. **Dubowitz scoring**

   Reflexes:
   - Stepping
   - Placing
   - Moro
   - Sucking
   - Rooting
   - Plantar grasp
   - Palmar grasp
   - Pincer grasp
   - APGAR Score.

Sign	*0*	*1*	*2*
Heart rate	Absent	Below 100	Over 100
Respiratory effort	Absent	Slow, irregular	Good, crying
Muscle tone	Limp	Some flexion of extremities	Active motion
Response to catheter in nostril (tested after oropharynx is clear)	No response	Grimace	Cough or sneeze
Color	Blue, pale	Body pink, extremities blue	Completely pink

NORMAL NEWBORN

1. **How will you measure the fontanelles?**
   i. Keep the tape on either side
   ii. Find the midpoint on both sides
   iii. Draw lines joining the opposite midpoints (line a / line b)

Anterior Fontanelle

Measure both 'a' and 'b'

$$\text{Length} = \frac{a+b}{2}$$

Normal: 2.5 cm
1.5 cm at 1 year

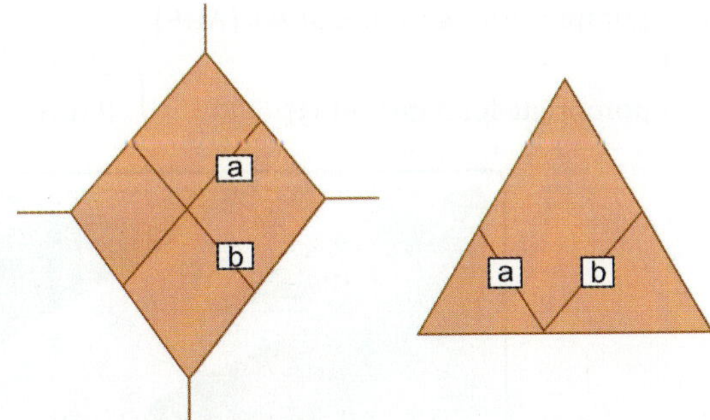

Posterior Fontanelle

Normal: 0.5–0.75 cm
Posterior fontanelle closes by 2–8 weeks.

2. **What are the features you infer by examining the newborns umbilical cord?**

Single umbilical artery → Ileal atresia, renal anomaly, genital anomaly and trisomy 18

Normal umbilical cord falls by 5–10 days (average: 7 days)

- Early fall → Sepsis
- Late fall → Factor XIII deficiency/ Lecithin—cholesterol acyltransferase (LCAT) deficiency

3. What do you infer when a newborn is edematous?

- Turner's syndrome → web neck, edema of dorsum of hands and feet
- Preterm → due to hypoproteinemia

4. How will you diagnose a child is having tracheoesophageal fistula from newborn period?

On examination: Drooling of saliva, frothy saliva

Diagnosed

- Large size 8 or 10 Fr plastic or gastric tube cannot be passed into as it gets arrested at 7–10 cm from mouth.
- Polythene catheter gets coiled up in the upper part of esophagus
- Accumulated secretions on aspiration is similar to gastric acid. But pH is not acidic.

X-ray Film

- Gas shadow in the stomach
  (Type I—where esophagus lower part connected to trachea)
- Lung shows atelectasis or pneumonia due to aspiration.

Can you suspect tracheoesophageal fistula from antenatal period?

Yes

- Maternal—polyhydramnios
- Birth single umbilical artery.

How will you measure head circumference? (Fig. 7.4)

Measure from external occipital protuberance to glabella

↓

Measurement at the point of parietal eminence

Classification

1. Appropriate for gestational age (AGF)
   (or)
   Appropriate for dates (AFD)
   } 2.5 kg
   'Birth weight between 10th to 90th percentile'

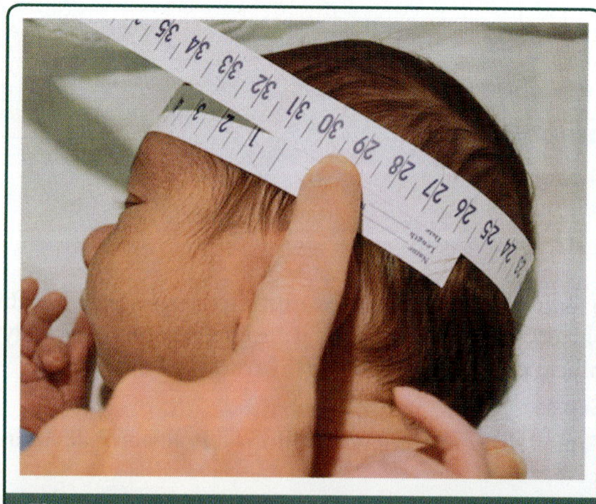

Figure: 7.4: Measurement of head circumference

2. SGA/SFD—< 2.5 kg (i.e) <10th percentile
3. LGA/LFD—>4.1 kg (i.e) >90th percentile

*SFA—Small for gestational age/dates
*LGA—Large for gestational age/dates

Growth Pattern

- First few days → Loses 10% body weight, i.e. about 3 kg = 300 g
- Next by age of 10 days → Regains the lost weight
- First 3 months → 25–35 g/day
- For first year

  Thereafter, i.e. 3–12 months → 400 g weight/month

  5 months → Doubles

  1 year → Triples

  2 years→ 4 times the birth weight
- Gains 2 kg/year → 3 to 7 years
- Gains 3 kg/year → until puberty.

Term

- Preterm—< 37 weeks
- Term—Between 37–42 weeks
- Post-term—> 42 weeks.

IUGR (SMALL FOR GESTATIONAL AGE)

Symmetrical (hypoplastic)	*Asymmetrical (malnourished)*
Insult has occurred in earlier part of gestation (1st trimester)	Insult has occurred in later part (2nd/3rd trimester)
Decrease in cell number Decrease in cell size	Decrease in cell size Not in number
All organs are affected—HC/AC/CC Decreased	HC will be normal other measurements decreased
When given food, takes long time to catch up growth	Catches up growth early

- But both types are prone for future attention deficits (learning abilities)
- Preterm has slow catch up but no future problem.

Features of Term Baby

- Ear lobes well-formed
- Breast nodules—5 mm
- Scrotal rugosities
- Testis descended
- External genitalia of female—majora covers minora.

Ponderal index: $\frac{\text{Wt (g)}}{\sqrt{\text{Ht (cm)}^3}} \times 100$

Average: 2

- <2: Asymmetrical IUGR
- >2: Symmetrical IUGR

CASE 1: PRETERM BABY

Causes

Socioeconomic

- Poor
- Poverty
- Illiteracy
- Illegitimacy
- Overcrowding
- Lower capita income
- Unwanted child

Maternal

- Anemia
- High risk:
  - Short stature: <145 cm
  - Weight less than: 40 kg
  - Hemoglobin <8 g
  - Age: <18 years and >35 years
- Bad obstetric history (BOH)
- Maternal sepsis : UTI, TB, renal, eclampsia/HTN/diabetes/trauma

Uterine Anomalies

- Bicornuate uterus
- Septate uterus
- Cervical incompetence
- Uterine myomas
- Hydramnios
- Vesicular moles
- Uterine infections
- Infarction
- Calcification
- TORCH agents
- Cord lesions: False/true knots

Baby Causes

- Multiple pregnancy
- Leg malformation
- Twin transfusion
- Chromosomal anomalies

Maternal Risk Factors

- Smoking
- Alcohol
- Hydantoin

Others

Iatrogenic: Improves diagnosis of maturity in cesarean deliveries.

Classification

LBW : <2.5 kg
High-risk LBW : <2 kg
Very low LBW : <1.5 kg
Extreme LBW : <1 kg

Prevention

1. Improve maternal nutrition
2. Rest
3. Fetal monitoring
4. Tocolytics
   - Isoxsuprie
   - Salbutamol
   - Terbutaline
5. Steroids: for lung maturity

   In unavoidable preterm:
   - Drug of choice: Betamethasone 12 mg in 2 doses
   - Dexamethasone can be given if associated with periventricular leukomalacia
6. Phenobarbitone in mother (Decrease incidence of jaundice and bleeding in fetus)
   - Single dose: 60 mg in mother

Discussion in Preterm Case

Preterm Infant

Features

- **General**: Hypotonia, extended posture
- **Skin:** Thin/blood vessels seen clearly with or without peripheral cyanosis
- **Ear lobes**: Decreased recoiling
- **Breast node**: <5 mm
- **Plantar crease**: Only deep crease seen faintly, superior crease not seen
- **Male child**: Undescended testis, decreased rugosities of scrotum
- **Female child**: Labia minora exposed

Handicaps in Preterm

It is the physiological immaturity in newborn which makes baby handicap.

I. **CNS:**

   1. **Intraventricular hemorrhage:** Because germinal layers are thin , characterized by pallor and convulsions resulting in spastic cerebral palsy, if they survive.

2. **Recurrent apneic attacks**: Because of immature brain stem and obstruction to airway.
3. **Hypothermia**: Immature thermal zone-shock/death.

II. CVS:
1. PDA
2. Pulmonary HTN
3. O_2 therapy causes:
   i. Persistent foramen ovale (PFO)
   ii. Pulmonary HTN
   iii. RS- pneumothorax
   iv. Bronchopulmonary dysplasia (BPD)
   v. Retrolental fibroplasias

III. Respiratory syndrome (RS)
1. Respiratory distress syndrome (RDS)
2. Hyaline membrane disease (HMD) (common <32 weeks)
3. Aspiration

IV. GIT:
1. Put IV fluids → Absent swallowing reflex if fed
   ↓
   Aspiration
2. Necrotizing enterocolitis
3. Prolonged physiological jaundice

V. General:
1. Sepsis (B cell immunity ↓)
2. Hypothermia
3. Electrolyte imbalance (↓ Na, ↓Ca, ↓Mg and glucose)
   ↓
   C/O Convulsions

Management

1. **Intraventricular hemorrhage**:
   - Maintain hydration
   - Vitamin K as a routine
   - Treat hypoxia

   Normal: Preterm—Vitamin K, 0.5 mg IM

   (Term—Vitamin K, 1 mg IM

   Even upto 10 mg to be given in the case of intraventricular hemorrhage.
2. **Hyaline membrane disease (HMD)**
   - Give steroids (dexamethasone before delivery)
   - X-ray
   - Treatment: Surfactant
3. **CVS:**
   - PDA
   - Indomethacin/ibuprofen (medical closure)
4. **Jaundice**: Phototherapy
5. **Sepsis**: Blood culture and sensitivity
6. **Metabolic disturbance**:

   Hypoglycemia: When blood glucose <45 mg/dL (Normal infants: <54 mg/dL)
   - 2 mL/kg 10% dextrose as a bolus
   - 5% Dextrose (babies <1 kg)

Hypocalcemia: Calcium gluconate 2 mL/kg, 10% calcium gluconate

Hyponatremia: Sodium chloride 2%

7. **Necrotizing enterocolitis:** (NEC)- also called as pigbel

   Causative organism—*Clostridium perfringens (Cl Welchii)*

   Babies very sick, hypothermic

   X-ray abdomen: Bowel distended
   - Lumen air shadow
   - Air under diaphragm

   Treatment:
   - Bowel rest
   - Replace electrolytes

Culture and sensitivity with appropriate antibiotics
Prevention: Weaning from IV fluids as early as possible.

CASE 2: NEONATAL JAUNDICE

Physiological Jaundice

	Appears in days	*Peak*	*Disappears in days*
Term	2	4–6	10
Preterm	2	7–9	14

Clinical assessment of jaundice level: Kramer's scale:

1. Face: 5 mg/dL
2. Chest: 10 mg/dL
3. Below umbilicus upto knee: 12 mg/dL
4. Upto feet: 15 mg/dL
5. Palms/soles: >15 mg/dL

Reasons for non-closure of posterior fontanelle in 1–2 weeks:

1. Hydrocephalus
2. Congenital hypothyroidism
3. Down's syndrome

Transcutaneous Bilirubinometer (T_CB)

- Direct reading by keeping over chest
- Gives the correct value even under phototherapy

Criteria for Physiological Jaundice

1. Appears after 48 hours
2. Peak 4–5 days
3. Disappears by 7–10 days
4. Never goes beyond 15 mg/dL
5. Preterm: Peak in 7 days/disappears by 10–14 days

Causes

1. Increase bilirubin load on liver—Increased erythrocyte volume, increased enterohepatic circulation, decreased RBC survival

2. Defective hepatic uptake of bilirubin from plasma
   (↓ ligandin
   ↑ Binding of ligandin by other anions
   ↓ Uptake in phase II)
4. Defective bilirubin conjugation (↓ UDPG activity)
5. Defective bilirubin excretion

Exaggeration of Physiological Jaundice

Causes

1. Congenital hypothyroidism (H/O coarse cry/abdomen distension/umbilical hernia)
2. Congenital pyloric stenosis (H/O vomiting/VGP/abdomen distension)
3. Infants with polycythemia
4. Infants of diabetic mothers
5. Delayed cord clamping
6. Breast milk jaundice
7. Congenital infections
8. Congenital heart disease

Criteria for Pathological Jaundice

1. Jaundice appearing in first 24 hours
2. Increase in total bilirubin level by more than 0.5 mg/dL/hr (or) 5 mg/dL/24 hr
3. Total bilirubin >15 mg/dL
4. Direct bilirubin >2 mg/dL

Causes

1. Erythroblastosis fetalis (Rh incompatibility) → manifests in first 12 hours, even as early as 30 minutes
2. ABO incompatibilty → After 12 hours
3. Hereditary spherocytosis
4. G6PD—deficiency, vitamin K_3 deficiency
5. Infection/sepsis
6. Pyloric stenosis (↑EHC)
7. Crigler-Najjar syndrome (I and II)
8. Hypothyroidism
9. Obstructive: Intrahepatic - Caroli's disease
   Extrahepatic - TORCH/infectious hepatitis

What is the difference between?

1. **Breast milk jaundice:**
   - 2nd week to 3rd month in exclusively breastfed infants
   - Due inhibitor substances in breast (pregnanediol, FFA)
   - Level >20 mg/dL attained

   #### *Treatment*

   Temporary cessation of breastfeeding

2. **Breastfeeding jaundice**:
   - Higher bilirubin level (peak) attained in first few days
   - Never seen in bottle-fed.

Treatment

Phototherapy: (370–420 nm)

Height: 45 centimeters

Types

1. Ordinary day light
2. Blue light (420–480 nm)
3. Green light

Principle

1. Geometric photoisomerization: Fat soluble bilirubin is converted to water-soluble component and excreted.
2. Structural isomerization:

   Bilirubin converted to lumirubin

   Excreted in bile without conjugation
3. Oxidation:

   To colorless products excreted by liver/kidney without conjugation

   Plexiglass is used to prevent UV radiation.

Types of Phototherapy (Fig. 7.5)

1. **Single**: One light source
2. **Double**: Two (each from either side)
3. **Triple**: Two from sides, one from below
4. **Spot**: Spot of light allowed to fall on chest (no need to cover eyes)
5. **Fibroptic**: (Biliblanket) Interwoven glass connected to (fiberoptic glass) light source.

Advantage is heat is not produced.

Treat water loss by 20–40 mL additional fluids

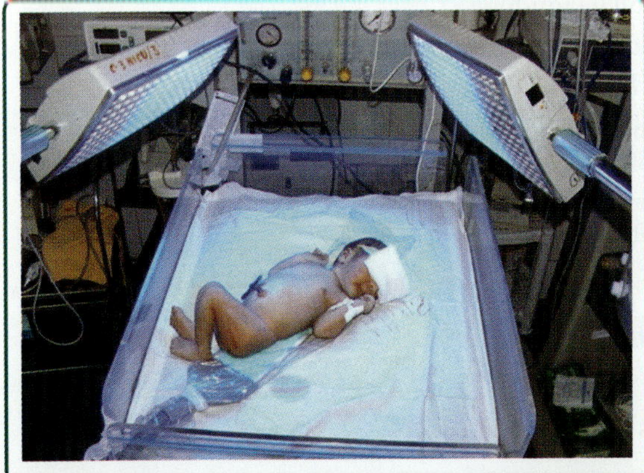

Figure 7.5: Phototherapy

Complications

1. Disturbance in eye: Retinal damage, lens coagulation, opacification
2. Water loss: Insensible loss
3. Genital damage

Long-term Effects

1. Disturbance of circadian rhythm (delayed menarche)
2. Chromosomal damage/mutation
3. Skin cancers

Contraindication

1. Direct hyperbilirubinemia → Bilirubin is converted to lumirubin (bronze baby syndrome)
2. Congenital erythropoietic purpura: Characterized by hemolysis/pink urine; Spleen + bullous skin lesions
3. Increased direct bilirubin
4. Idiopathic thrombocytopenic purpura.

Where will you give prophylactic phototherapy?

1. Extremely LBW
2. Awaiting exchange transfusion
3. ABO incompatibility
4. Severely bruised

Types of Phototherapy

- Continuous
- Intermittent
- Prophylactic

Exchange Transfusion

Ideal blood group: Mother blood group

1. Push and pull technique
2. Exchange double volume(160 mL/kg body weight in 2 hours)
3. 60% pre exchange level

Ideal blood groups to be used:
Rh incompatibility:

- Rh negative; ABO compatible blood

ABO incompatibility:

- O group; Rh compatible

Complications

1. Infection
2. Thrombosis (portal vein)
3. Umbilical
4. Arrhythmias, cardiac arrest

5. Embolism
6. Electrolyte imbalance: Decreased magnesium, calcium, hypoglycemia, academia and alkalosis.

   During each push and pull technique—use only 5–10 mL.

Monitor

Bilirubin and electrolyte level after transfusion.

Precautions during phototherapy:

1. Damage can occur to fastly multiplying cells in retina and testis
2. Cover the retina and testis.

Viva: What is the adverse effect you expect in preterm babies given phototherapy?
Patency of Ductus Arteriosus
↓
While discharging the baby check for continuous murmur at 2nd ICS at time of discharge
Prevention:
By keeping a tin sheet over 2nd ICS

Disadvantages of O_2 therapy in future

1. Retrolental fibroplasias
2. Bronchopulmonary dysplasia
3. Persistent foramen ovale in atrial septum.

Surgical causes of jaundice in newborn

1. Biliary atresia
2. Choledochal cyst (congenital dilatation of biliary system)
3. Pyloric stenosis.

Viva Discussion

Causes of infection in newborn (preterm)

1. Maternal antibodies not transferred properly
2. Lymphnode is not formed which controls infection
3. Decreased IgG immune system maturation
4. Immunological memory not formed (recognition of infection previously affected).

Why should you need not breastfed in preborn (<34 weeks)?

1. Swallowing reflex—not established
2. Sphincter not yet became tight
3. Cough reflex not yet established
4. Coordination not yet obtained.

How will you feed IUGR infant?
Expressed breast milk.

Fed in the following ways:

1. Katori (paladai)
2. Gavage
3. Drip method

4. Nasojejunal feeding
5. Nasogastric feeding
6. Parenteral feeding:
   - Dextrose
   - IV fluids
   - Blood products
   - PPN (partial parenteral nutrition)
   - TPN (total parenteral nutrition)

Treatment of Newborn

1. Thermal treatment
2. Fluid treatment
3. Infection

Thermoneutral Environment

Two types of temperature: Core temperature (34–35°C), skin temperature (0.5°C less than core temperature), <36°C—hypothermia

Prevention of hypothermia:
10 steps of warm chain:
1. Warm delivery room
2. Warm resuscitation
3. Immediate drying
4. Skin to skin contact between baby and mother
5. Breastfeeding
6. Postponement of bathing
7. Rooming in
8. Bedding in warm
9. Warm transport
10. Training of healthcare providers

Preterm baby:

i. Skin is very thin due to absence of subcutaneous fat
ii. Keeps the limbs extended
iii. If he has hypothermia, he does not cry so lose the temperature

Normal temperature:

Term	*Preterm*
1. Skin is thick due to subcutaneous fat	Thin
2. Keep the limbs closed	Extended
3. If hypothermia present, it cries, so there is increased temperature	Absent cry
4. Shivering is present	Absent
5. Brown pad of fat is present over the adrenals (Increased mitochondria, increased blood supply)	Brown pad of fat is absent

Methods of maintaining temperature:

Treatment of Hypothermia

1. Cover the baby with towel, plastic cover to cover Very Low Birth Weight (VLBW) babies in emergency
2. Rooming in (natural incubator)
3. Kangaroo mother care
4. Two-layered cotton to be closed with coconut oil over baby for treatment and transfer
5. 200 watts bulb over 2 feet height in houses
6. Villages—keep the windows closed; Burning charcoal without smoke
7. Warmers

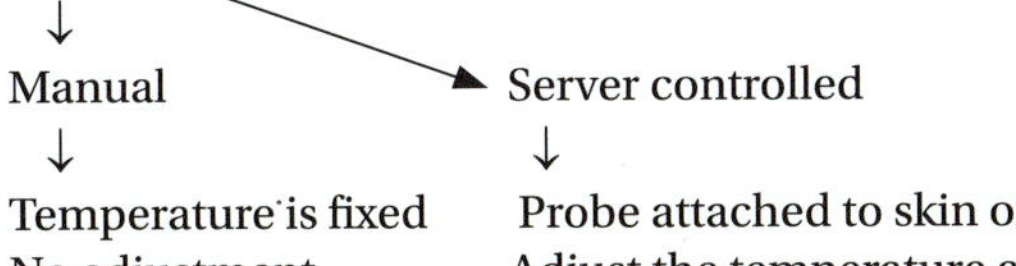

8. Room heaters can be kept.

Fluid Management

Newborn: Normal: 60–80 mL/kg
Increased up to 140 mL/kg
Preterm: May go upto 80–100 mL/kg

Investigations

1. **Gastric aspirate**: Count the leukocytes
   >2 : Sepsis
   <2 : Normal

   Sepsis screening:
   1. Micro ESR
   2. Absolute neutrophil count
   3. Platelet count
   4. Immature neutrophils band ratio

2. **Blood sample**: TC, DC
   Micro ESR: 4 mm in infection
   NEC: Decreased
   Toxic granules
3. **Swab**: Umbilicus, Pustules, Ear/nose/throat } Gram-negative sepsis, Group B beta-hemolytic Streptococci
4. **X-ray**: Paralytic ileus, pneumonic consolidation
5. **Urine/Blood/CSF**: C/S

Treatment of Infections

Higher antibiotics: Ampicillin + cefatoxime (3rd generation)
- Penicillin (broad coverage)
- Cefatoxime + gentamicin

If very sick: Blood transfusion
- Exchange transfusion

CASE 3: IUGR (INTRAUTERINE GROWTH RESTRICTION) INFANT

Small for Gestational Age (SGA)

Birth weight less than 10th percentile are called SGA or small for dates (SFD).

Causes

I. **Maternal**: Short stature
   - Primi/grand multipara
   - Young mother
   - Fetal alcohol/hydantoin syndrome
   - Anemia, heart disease
   - Preeclampsia, hypertension

II. **Fetal:** Chromosomal anomalies
   - Multiple pregnancies
   - Intrauterine infections

III. **Placental:** Abruptio placenta
   - Placenta previa
   - Placental infarcts
   - Bicornuate/septate uterus

Clinical features of IUGR:
- Old man face
- Loose skin
- Thin subcutaneous fat
- Post dated/low birth weight

Classification

Ponderal Index

- >2: Symmetrical IUGR
- <2: Asymmetrical IUGR
- **Symmetrical**: Size of head is reduced proportional to body
- **Asymmetrical**: Size of head is large as compared to body.
  - HC - CC = >3 cm.
  - (Normal: 3 cm) Here >3 cm

Symmetrical IUGR: It is due to intrauterine infections and it catches up the growth very slowly on feeding.

Complications of IUGR Baby

Meconium Aspiration Syndrome

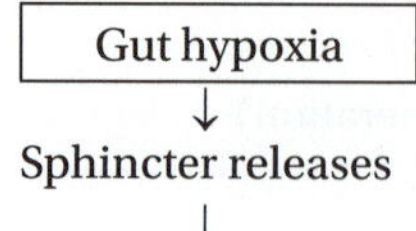

Meconium released into amniotic fluid because of gasping respiration

Aspirates meconium
↓
Pneumonia
atelectasis ← enters bronchioles
Collapse
Emphysema
↓
Progressed to air leak syndromes

I. Pneumothorax
II. Pneumopericardium
III. Pneumomediastinum

- The meconium → chemical pneumonitis
- Think meconium → Atelectasis, emphysema air leak syndromes

Hypothermia

- Decreased brown pad of fat
- Large surface area → more evaporation, conduction and convention
- Decreased muscular activity

Infection/thrombocytopenia

Hypoxia → Erythropoietic series increased production
↓
Compensatory decreased production of platelets/neutrophils
↓
Infection

Hypoglycemic

Small baby →

i. ↓ Glycogen storage
ii. ↓ Glucose production
iii. ↓ Glycogenolysis

C/F related to release of adrenaline and ANS activation

- Sweating
- Tremors
- Jitteriness—symmetrical movement—earliest sign
- Apnea
- Convulsions
- Bradycardia

Bleeding manifests

(Polycythemia/hyperviscosity)

- Vitamin K dependent factors are not synthesized adequately → bleeding manifests
- Tissue thromboplastin release → disseminated intravascular coagulation (DIVC)

Polycythemia → increased erythropoietin → DIVC
↓

Thrombosis in

i. Cerebral veins → convulsions
ii. Renal vein thrombosis → Renal mass palpable
iii. Pulmonary apoplexy → sudden pulmonary hemorrhage

Ossification Decreased

Anterior fontanelle large

Congenital Malformations

Common among hypoplastic

Investigations

- X-ray
- PCV: 40–60 (normal) >60% = hyperviscosity
- Serum electrolytes
- R/O Infections

Treatment

- If PCV >60% = Partial exchange transfusion (with normal saline)

$$\text{Amount to be transfused} = \frac{(\text{Observed hematocrit} - \text{Derived hematocrit}) \times 100}{\text{Volume of blood}}$$

Treat the Complications

- 10% dextrose IV 2 mL/kg body weight for hypoglycemia
- Meconium aspiration syndrome: Chemical pneumonitis
  - Antibiotics → To prevent infection
  - O_2 administered
  - IV fluids
  - Steroid (minimal use)
- Radiant warmers: For hypothermia
- Kangaroo mother care

Kangaroo Mother Care

- Keeping the baby in skin to skin contact with mother/caregiver
- No risk of hyperthermia/temperature swing
- Based on thermal synchrony principle:
  - Constant temperature maintained at 37°C
  - If baby's temperature is decreased by 1°C, mother's body temperature increases by 2°C
  - If baby's temperature is increased by 1°C, mother's body temperature is decreased by 1°C
- Keep the baby in between the breast in a frog-like position with head semiflexed/laterally without cloth except caps and socks
- Indicated for all stable low birth weight (LBW) babies, less than 1.8 kg.

Reflexes in Newborn

Neonatal Reflexes			
Moro reflex	Hold infant in supine position; support head and neck with hand; allow head to drop while still supporting it	Spreading: Arms abduct, extend; hands open Hugging: Arms adduct and flex; hands close	Unequal laterality Absence of spread; Asymmetry; Exaggeration with disorganization in state
Tonic neck reflex	Infant in supine, neutral position; turn head to one side; repeat opposite side;	Mental extension, occipital flexion; primarily of arms; does not remain in position for >30 seconds	Exaggerated response and stays in position >30 seconds
Withdrawal reflex	Painful stimulus to one foot	Withdrawal of stimulated foot; variable extension of opposite leg	Absence of flexion in stimulated leg
• ATNR, asymmetric tonic neck reflex (Fig. 3.1) • Persistence beyond this, is abnormal – Palmar grasp (3–4 months) – Moro reflex (5 months) – Asymmetric tonic reflex (6 months) – Plantar grasp (9–12 months)			

Other reflexes:

1. Pierre reflex:

   pressure over spine

   ↓

   Flexion of both the lower limbs

2. Galen Reflex:

   Pressure over paravertebral region, i.e stroke over R/L side of the paravertebral region

   ↓

   Extension of that side R/L limb.

CASE 8 Spotters

SPOTTER 1: HYDROCEPHALUS (FIG. 8.1)

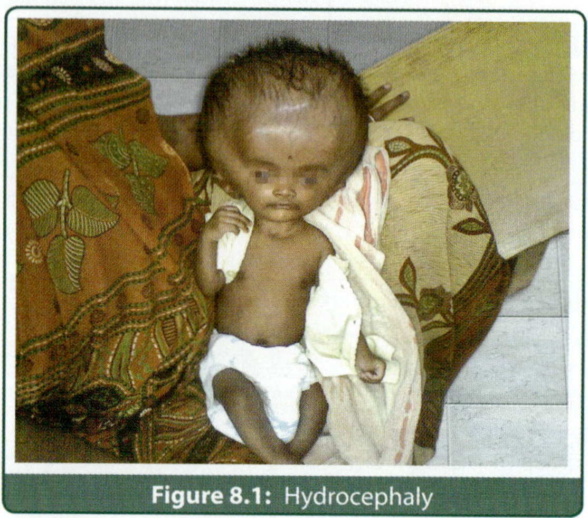

Figure 8.1: Hydrocephaly

Pathophysiology of CSF (Fig. 8.2)

By plasma ultrafiltration and active secretion.

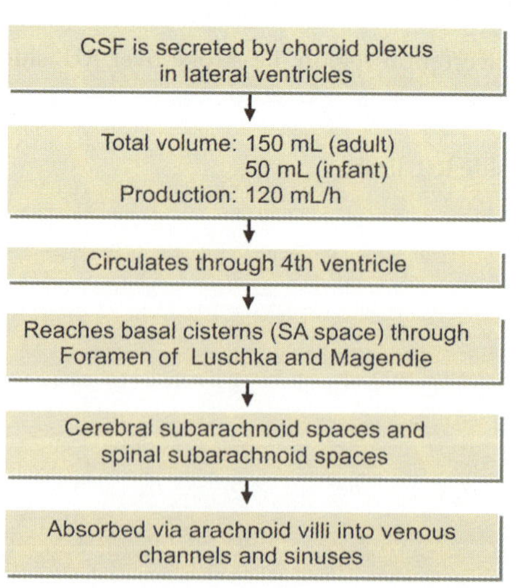

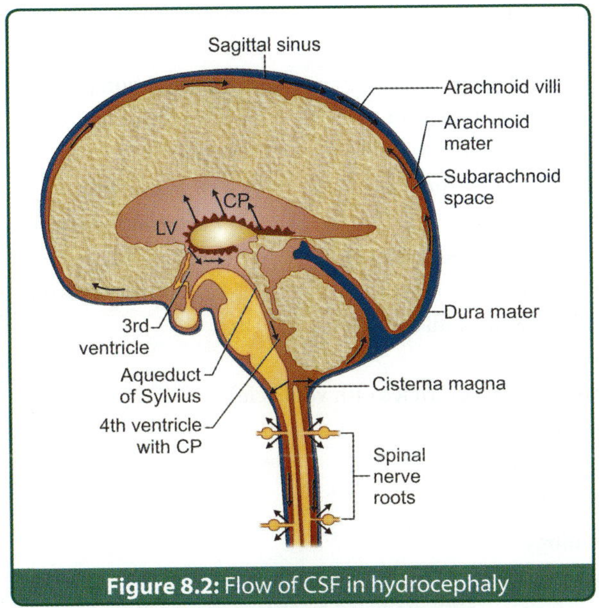

Figure 8.2: Flow of CSF in hydrocephaly

Types of Hydrocephalus

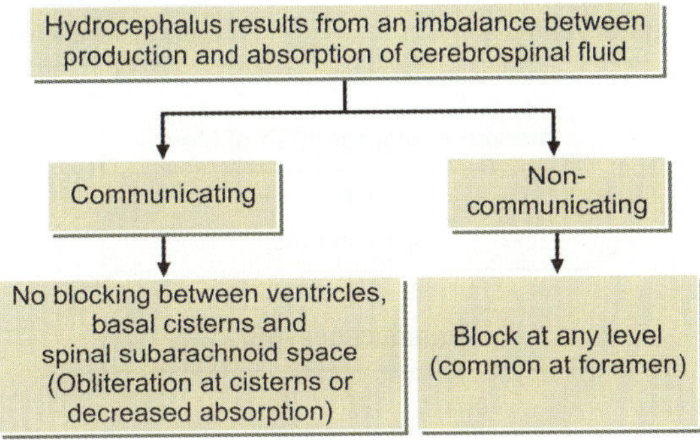

ETIOLOGY

Congenital

1. **Aqueductal stenosis**
   (X-linked recessive)
   Due to intrauterine infections like toxoplasmosis
2. **Arnold-Chiari malformation**:
   (Downward displacement of cerebellum with brainstem

Acquired

1. **Obstructive:**
   Congenital malformations
   Tumor
   Periaqueductal stenosis
   Cystic lesions
   Fibrosis
   Intraventricular hemorrhage (m/c)
   (Ventricles above obstruction is dilated—DD from communicating)
2. **Communicating:**
   Follows
   Chronic meningitis

into cervical canal)

Commonest type 2 Chiari malformation, cerebellum and medulla are shifted caudally with distortion and obstruction of CSF pathway (associated with meningomyelocele)

3. **Posterior fossa cyst:**
   (Dandy-Walker malformation)
   Posterior fossa cyst
   Communicating with ventricles (4th ventricle)
4. **Intrauterine infections:**
   Intracranial bleeds
   Congenital tumors

Meningoencephalitis
↓
↑ Production at choroid space
↓ Absorption at subarachnoid space
- TB meningitis
- Posterior fossa tumors
- Ruptured aneurysm
- Post-intraventricular hemorrhage

Pathophysiology

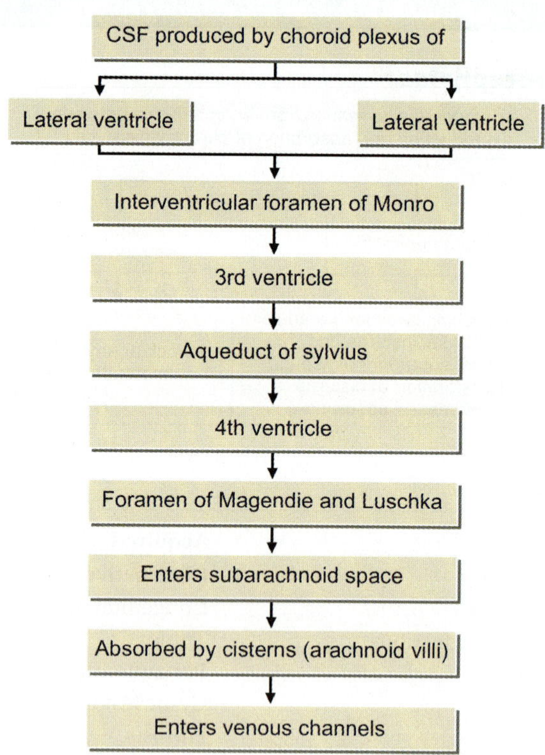

Hydrocephalus is due to
- Increased production
- Decreased absorption
- Any obstruction

Clinical Features

- **Macrocephalus**: More than 2.5 cm, i.e. >2 SD above the mean for that age, i.e. {1SD = 1.25 cm} (Fig. 8.3)
- **Fontanelle**: Remains open
- **Sutures**: Delayed closure
- **Shiny scalp veins/brow bulges:**

1. Crackpot/Macewen's sign: Due to wide open fontanelle.
2. Sunset sign: Dilated ventricles push the supraspinal recess (Fig. 8.4) → Presses on tectum ↓ On eyeball ↓ Upper sclera visible
3. Transillumination positive (Dark room test)
   - >5–8 mm: Significant in forehead
   - >10 mm: Significant in occiput

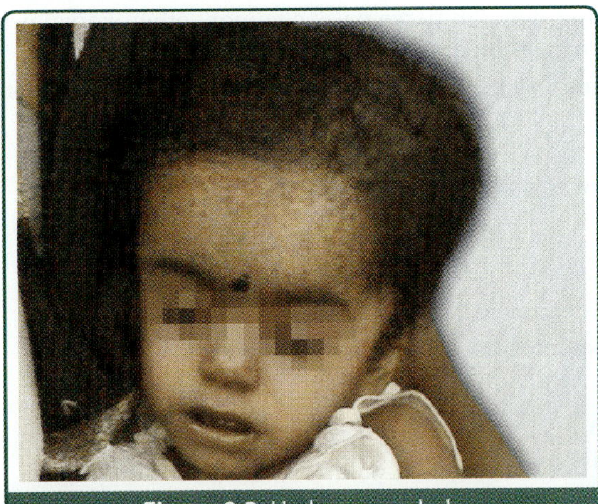

Figure 8.3: Hydranencephaly

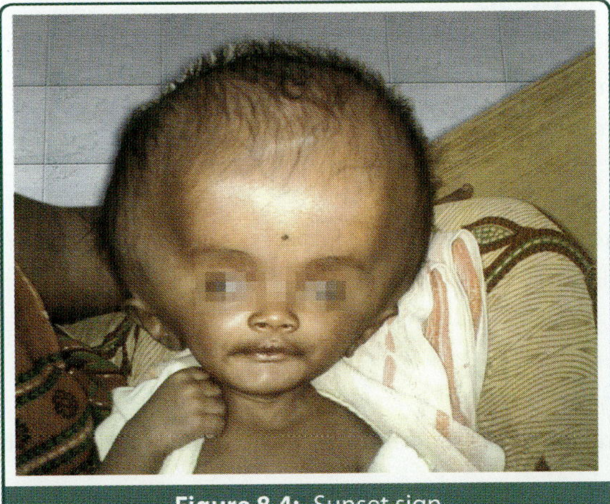

Figure 8.4: Sunset sign

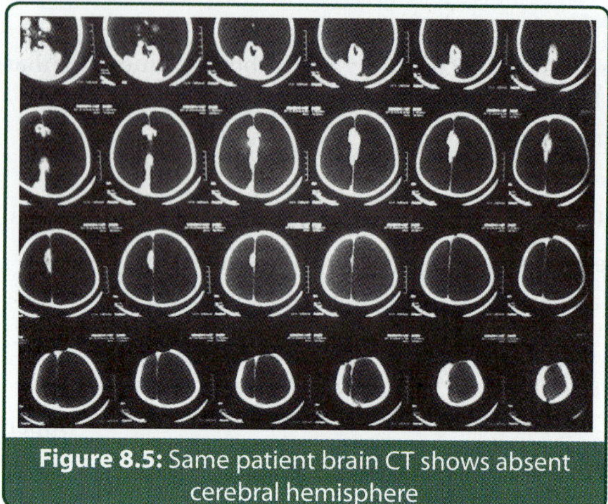

Figure 8.5: Same patient brain CT shows absent cerebral hemisphere

On Examination

1. **False localizing sign:** 6th nerve palsy common, other cranial nerve may also be involved (though lesion not at brainstem, 6th palsy is seen).
2. **Increased tone/brisk tendon jerks**: Due to compression of white matter (lower limb more).

Features of Increased ICT

1. Papilledema
2. Ophthalmoplegia
3. Bradycardia (decreased heart rate (HR))
4. Abnormal respiratory rate (RR)/Rhythm—increased
5. Constipation
6. Optic atrophy
7. Blurring of disc
8. False localizing sign

Differential Diagnosis

1. Macrocephaly
2. Megalencephaly
3. Neurocutaneous syndrome
4. Familial large head
5. Subdural effusion
6. Achondroplasia
7. Hemolytic anemias
8. Rickets

Investigations

I. **Cranial ultrasound**: Screen ventricles or subdural space through provided open fontanelle.

II. CT scan: Ventricles size (Fig. 8.5)
Periventricular ooze (indication of increased ventricular pressure)
Thickness of cortical mantle
Coexisting lesions
Possible etiology

X-ray—beaten silver appearance: Hydrocephalus developing after closure of sutures result in sutural diastasis and convolutional markings of brainstem.

Treatment

Medical management: Acetazolamide 50 mg/kg/day; Glycerol
Surgical management: Ventriculoperitoneal/ventriculoatrial shunts
Complications of VP shunt:

- *Staphylococcus albus* infection
- Infective endocarditis
- Obstruction
- Arrhythmias

Complications

1. Optic nerve atrophy
2. Cerebral diplegia (lower leg fibers)
3. 6th nerve palsy
4. Increased intracranial tension

Osteogenesis Imperfecta

It can cause hydrocephalus by obstruction of improper bone in CSF tract
↓
H/O - Multiple fractures
O/E - Blue sclera
Tell one more condition where you get multiple fractures?
Battered baby syndrome (BBS)
(Take X-ray of other limb above, if has fracture similar to this limb, it is a case of sure Battered baby syndrome).

Other Features of Hydrocephalus

Hydrocephalus Ex vacuo

- In cerebral atrophy, ventricles are dilated but pressure not raised.

Differential Diagnosis

1. Rickets: Frontal bossing (philosopher's head)
   - Large head
   - Size of head within normal for age
   - Suture not separated
   - Other rachitic signs
2. A large dolicocephalic head
3. Familial large head (**megalencephaly**) no signs of ICT

4. Rapidly increasing size of head of premature infants (do serial measurements of head circumference)
5. Achondroplasia: Anterior fontanelle/sutures—normal
6. Hurler's syndrome: Large head
7. Subdural hematoma:
   - Square top
   - In biparietal diameter
   - H/O trauma

   C/O: Restlessness
   Vomiting
   Failure to thrive
   Convulsion
   Neck stiffness
8. Hydroencephaly:
   - Cerebral hemispheres not developed
   - Thin cortex large ventricle

   Differential diagnosis: Transillumination
9. Thickened cranium: Hemolytic anemia
   - Osteogenesis imperfecta
   - Rickets
   - Epiphyseal dysplasia
10. Metabolic/degenerative disorder of CNS:
    - Tay-Sachs disease
    - Maple syrup urine disease
    - Leukodystrophies.

Diagnosis

H/O:

1. Familial 'X' linked (Aqueductal stenosis)
2. Café au lait spots
3. Past H/O meningitis, mumps encephalitis
4. Occiput prominent → Dandy; occiput foreshortened → Chiari
5. Serial HC measurement
6. Anterior fontanelle not closed
7. Cranial bruit: Galen arteriovenous malformation
8. Cerebellar tonsil + Dandy-Walker: Massive dilatation
9. Chorioretintis: Toxoplasma
10. Papilledema: Rare due to separation of sutures due to increased intracranial tension.

SPOTTER 2: DOWN'S SYNDROME (LANGDON SYNDROME)

→ Trisomy - 21
→ Mongolism

- Risk of recurrence:
  - Mother carrier—10%
  - Father carrier—5%
- Commonest chromosomal disorder
- Present in triplicate

Incidence: 1 in 800 live births

Extrachromosomal is maternal always. Why?
Maternal oocyte is exposed to harmful environmental influences for a longer period, since follicles are present from fetal life while sperm has a shorter lifespan.

Complaints and Past History

- Delayed milestones
- Delayed passage of meconium
- Recurrent vomiting
- Prolonged jaundice
- Recurrent respiratory tract
- Feeding difficulties: Cleft lip, palate
- Did baby still lie for long time periods? (congenital hypothyroidism)

Head to foot examination (Figs 8.6 to 8.8):

1. **Skull (Fig. 8.8):**
   - Brachycephalic
   - Flat occiput
   - Opened anterior fontanelle/persistent posterior fontanelle
   - Low hair line
   - Sparse hair

   Plagiocephaly: Asymmetrical head on one side
   Scaphocephaly (also called dolichocephaly): Boat-shaped (AP diameter increased due to premature closure of sagittal fissure)
   Brachycephaly: Decreased AP diameter
   Oxycephaly/Turricephaly: Tower-shaped head

2. **Eyes:**
   - Mongoloid slant (upward)
   - Prominence of medial epicanthal folds (pseudohypertelorism)
   - Refractory error/cataract
   - Nystagmus
   - White spot on iris: Brushfield spots in light skin people

3. **Nose:**
   - Flattened nasal bridge

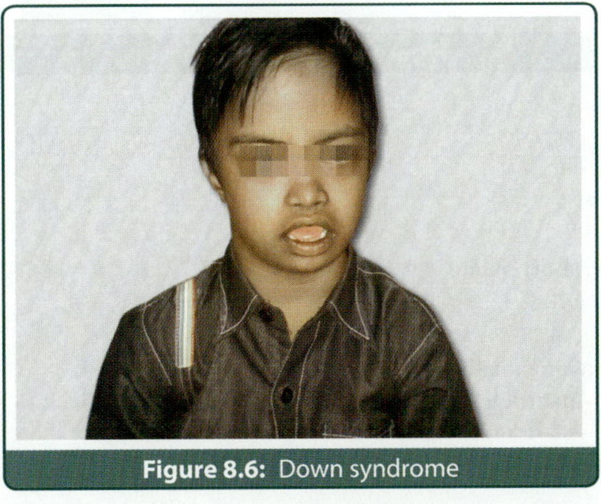

Figure 8.6: Down syndrome

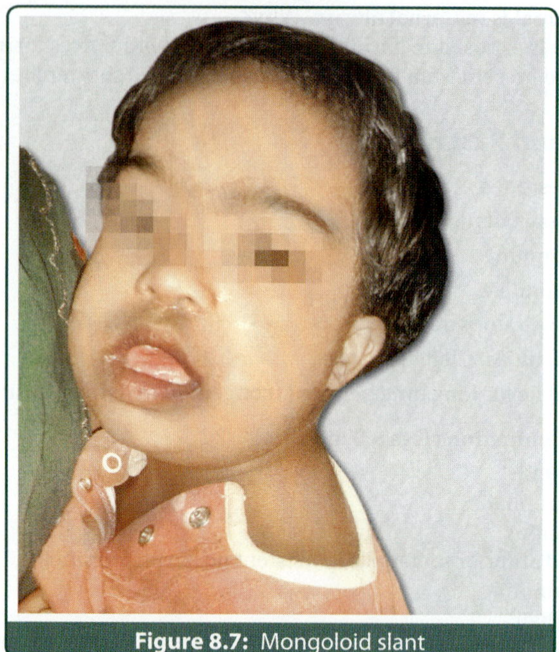

Figure 8.7: Mongoloid slant

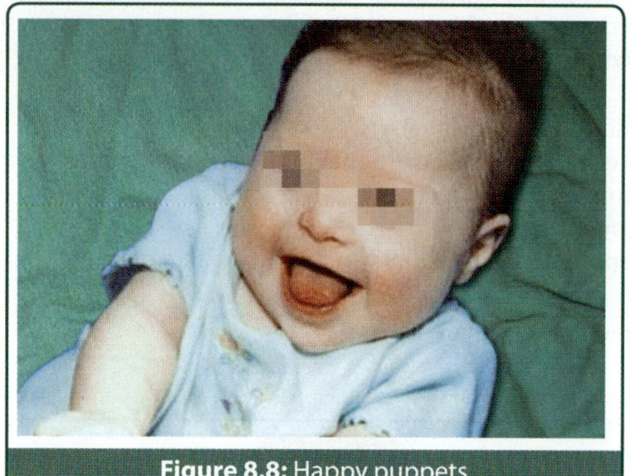

Figure 8.8: Happy puppets

4. **Ear:**
   - Low set ears
   - Deafness
5. **Mouth:**
   - Narrow, short palate
   - Small teeth
6. **Tongue:**
   - Hypoplastic maxilla
   - Pseudo-macroglossia because of hypoplasia → falls back → aspiration

     ↓

     Protruded outwards → fissured scrotal tongue

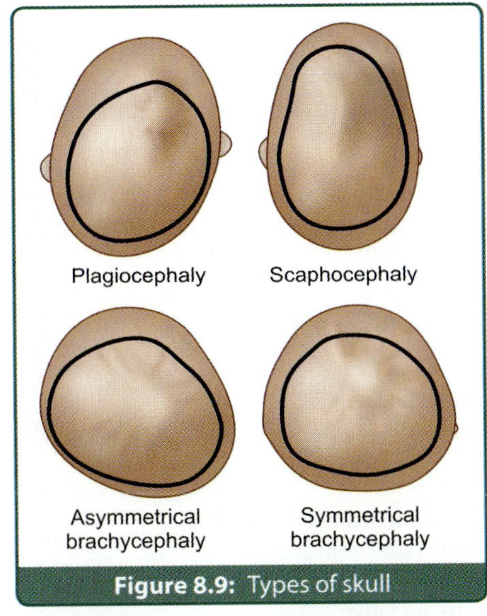

Figure 8.9: Types of skull

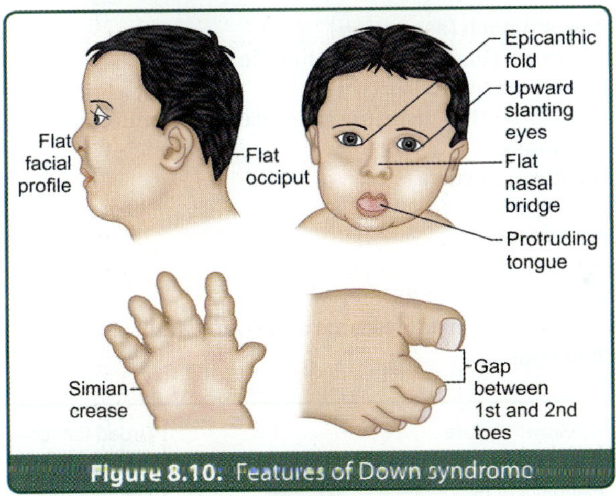

Figure 8.10: Features of Down syndrome

7. **Neck - short:**

   Skin: Loose folds of skin in nape of the neck

   1. Cutis marmorata } Early infancy
      Acrocyanosis of extremities
   2. Hyperkeratotic areas in wrist, elbow, knees
   3. Angular stomatitis

8. **Hand (Fig. 8.10):**
   - Short stubby fingers
   - Single palmar crease **(simian crease)**
   - Clinodactyly: Hypoplasia of middle phalanx with a single flexion crease of 5th finger (inward curving)
   - Typical dermatoglyphics
   - Distal triradius (junction of thenar, hypothenar and palmar dermal ridges)
   - More ulnar loops on fingers

9. **Abdomen:**
   - Protuberant (hypotonia)
   - Umbilical hernia
10. **Genitalia:**
    - Hypoplastic penis
    - Cryptorchidism
11. **Foot (Fig. 8.9):**
    - Gap between great toe and 2nd toe increased (Sandal gap)
    - Rocker bottom feet

Systemic Examination (Fig. 8.11)

1. **CVS:**
   Endocardial cushion defect:
   - ASD (ostium primum)
   - VSD
   - PDA

   What develops from endocardial cushion?
   - Upper part of ventricular septum
   - Lower part of atrial septum
   - Mitral valve, tricuspid valve
2. **GIT:**
   - Imperforate stomach (aspiration)
   - Duodenal atresia (Barium: double bubble)
     Annular pancreas
   - Imperforate anus (Hirschsprung's disease-like manifestation)
3. **Urogenital anomalies:**
   - Meconium through vulva
4. **CNS:**
   - Mental retardation
   - Hypotonia
   - Alzheimer's disease after 25–30 years
   - Reactive depression in adolescents and young adult
   - Autistic behavior

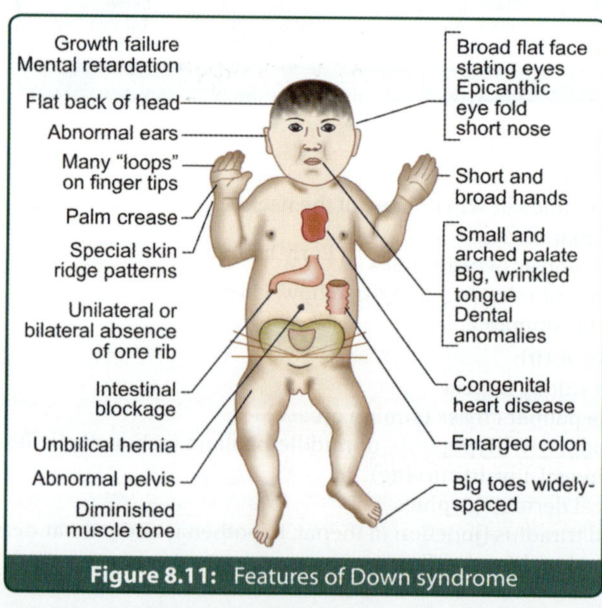

Figure 8.11: Features of Down syndrome

5. **Immune system:**
   - Frequent infection
   - Autoimmune diseases
   - Trace element deficiencies
6. **Endocrine problems:**
   - Congenital hypothyroidism
   - Girls—fertile; Boys—sterile
7. **Orthopedic problem:**
   - Joint laxity
   - Patella and hip dislocation
   - Atlantoaxial dislocation
8. **Hematological system:**
   - Acute leukemia
   - Congenital thrombocytopenia
   - Neonatal jaundice
   - Philadelphia chromosome positive in Down's syndrome

Causes of Trisomy 21

- Non-disjunction (older mother): 95%
- Translocation (younger mother)
  (G-G or D-G) Robertsonian 4%
  ↓
  can occur only between acrocentric chromosomes
- Mosaic type: 1% (mitotic non-disjunction)- good prognosis
  Presence of greater than 2 cell lines

Types of translocations:

- 14, 21
- 13, 21
- 15, 21
- 21, 21

Age of mother	*Risk*
15–29	1.1550
30–34	1:800
35–39	1:270
40–44	1:100
More than 45	1:50

Down syndrome in subsequent live births:

Type	*Parent carrying balanced translocation- Risk % in offspring*
14/21	Mother: 10% Father: 2.5% Neither parent: <1%
21/21	100%

What is the cause of sudden death in Down syndrome?

- Atlantoaxial joint dislocation
- **M/c cause of death: cardiac cause and infection**

Investigations

1. X-ray pelvis:
   - Shallow acetabular root
   - Flaring of ileum: Elephant ear-like ilium
   - Small sacroiliac notch
2. X-ray chest:
   - Eleven ribs
3. Chromosomal study: Buccal smear
4. Investigations of associated anomalies

Treatment

- No definite treatment
- Physiotherapy
- Early stimulation program
- Speech therapy in older children

Mongols are good babies and happy children, friendly. Have a good sense of rhythm and enjoy music. Hence, are called as happy puppets.

Causes of mortality and morbidity:

- Congenital heart disease (m/c)
- Chronic rhinitis, conjunctivitis, periodontal disease
- Lower respiratory tract infections
- Juvenile type of CML

Prognosis

- 80% survive beyond 30 years

Differential Diagnosis

1. **Cretinism:**
   - Large forehead
   - Coarse facial features
   - Rough hair
   - Altered cry
   - Hormonal assay: Abnormal
2. **Mucopolysaccharidosis (MPS)**
   - Coarse ugly facial features
   - Hepatosplenomegaly
   - MPS deposits
3. **Atonic cerebral palsy:**
   - Brisk reflexes

Prenatal Diagnosis of Down Syndrome

1. At risk pregnancy:
   - Mother age >35 years
   - Previous child with Down syndrome
2. Maternal serum marker: (Triple test/quadruple test)
   - Alpha fetoprotein: Decreased in 14–16 weeks
   - Unconjugated estriol: Decreased in 14–16 weeks
   - Human chorionic gonadotropin: Increased in 14–16 weeks
   - Pregnancy associated placental protein: Increased in 1st trimester
3. Amniocentesis (16th week)
4. Cordocentesis (18–20 weeks)
5. Chorionic villus sampling (9–11 weeks): Early to detect Down syndrome
6. Ultrasonogram:
   - Increased nuchal thickness (increased fatty deposit in the nape of neck)
   - Double bubble in abdomen
   - Short femur
   - Clinodactyly
   - Macroglossia
7. Fetal Echo: Endocardial cushion defect
8. Fetal cells in maternal circulation:
   - FISH-Focused in situ hybridization technique

SPOTTER 3: MICROCEPHALY (FIGS 8.12 AND 8.13)

Head circumference <3 SD for the mean age and sex and race (1 SD = 1.25 cm)

Causes

- Craniostenosis
- Poor development of brain

Types

1. Primary causes:
   - Familial: Normal mental development
   - Syndromes:
     - Smith-Lemli-Opitz syndrome
     - Rubinstein Taybi syndrome
     - Cornelia de Lange syndrome
2. Secondary causes:
   - Chromosomal anomalies:
     - Trisomy 13, 18,21
     - Cri-du-chat syndrome (5p deletion)
   - Congenital intrauterine infections (TORCH)
   - Irradiation during antenatal period
   - Maternal intake of drugs during pregnancy, fetal alcohol syndrome and fetal hydantoin syndrome
   - Hypoxic ischemic encephalopathy
   - Hyperthermia during pregnancy
   - Maternal malnutrition

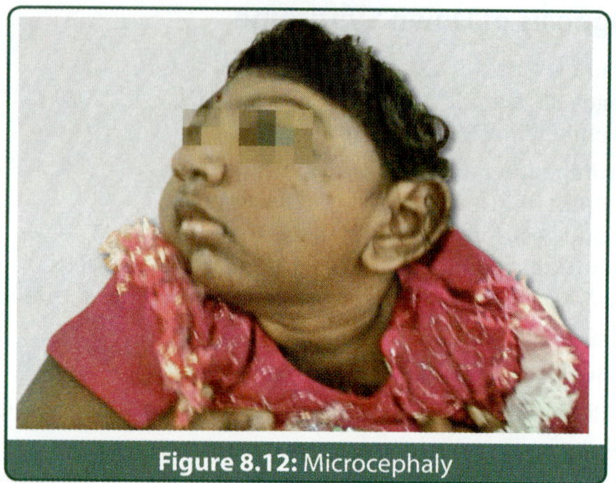

Figure 8.12: Microcephaly

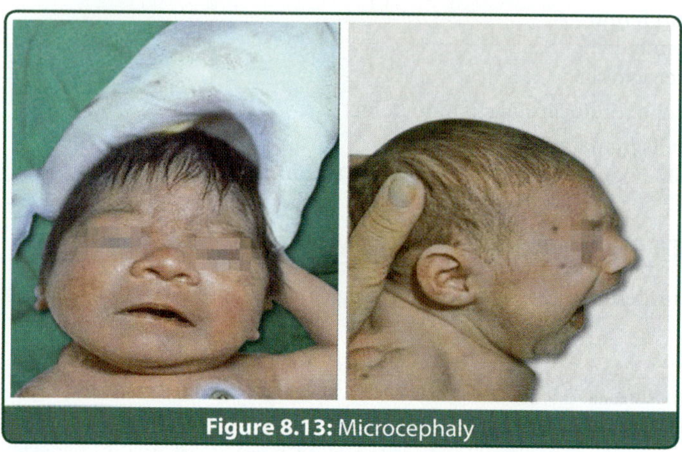

Figure 8.13: Microcephaly

Craniostenosis

(Premature closure of sutures) (Fig. 8.14)

Dolichocephaly (scaphocephaly)/ brachycephaly and plagiocephaly	*Microcephaly*
Anterior fontanelles closed	Anterior fontanelle open
Sutures are closed	Sutures not yet closed completely

Other Possible Spotters in Examination

1. **Phrynoderma—Toad skin (Fig. 8.15):**
   - Presence of small macules on the extensor surface of the elbow
   - Look for Bitot's spots in eyes also
   - Due to essential fatty acid deficiency
   - Vitamin A deficiency (most common)
   - Treatment:

     Vitamin A: 2 lakh IU on day 1 and 2; 3rd dose on 4th–6th week
     Ginger oil application on the lesion/also to drink

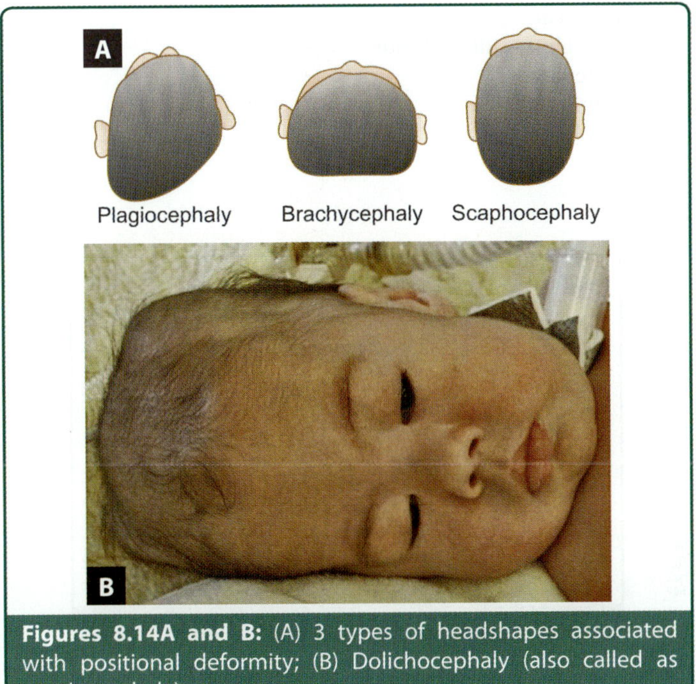

Figures 8.14A and B: (A) 3 types of headshapes associated with positional deformity; (B) Dolichocephaly (also called as scaphocephaly)

2. **Bitot's spots (Fig. 8.16)** Bitot's spots:
   - Due to vitamin A deficiency
3. **Scabies (Fig. 8.17)**:
   - Caused by *Sarcoptes scabiei*
   - Characterized by vesicles, papules with burrow in interdigital spaces, groin, elbow and axilla
   - Complications: Impetigo and acute glomerulonephritis
   - Treatment:
     Sulfur precipitate
     Benzyl benzoate: 2% solution
     Permethrin 1%
     Gamma benzene hexachloride (BHC)
     - Apply below neck throughout
     - Treat all family members
     - Wash the infected materials separately
4. **Impetigo:**
   - Two types: Bullous and Non-bullous impetigo
   - Bullous—caused by *Staphylococcus aureus*: Appears as yellow pustules
   - Non-bullous—caused by beta-hemolytic *Streptococci*: Appears as yellow crusts
   - Complications:
     Staphylococcal
     - Cellulitis
     - Osteomyelitis
     - Septic arthritis
     - Pneumonia
     - Septicemia

Streptococcal
- Acute glomerulonephritis
- Scarlet fever
- Lymphangitis
- Lymphadenitis

Color Plate:

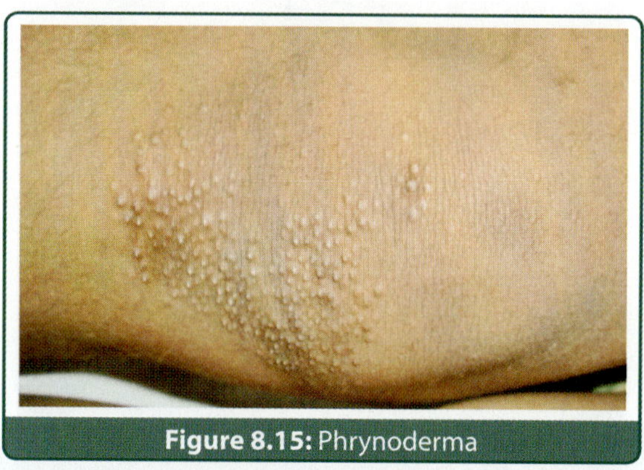

Figure 8.15: Phrynoderma

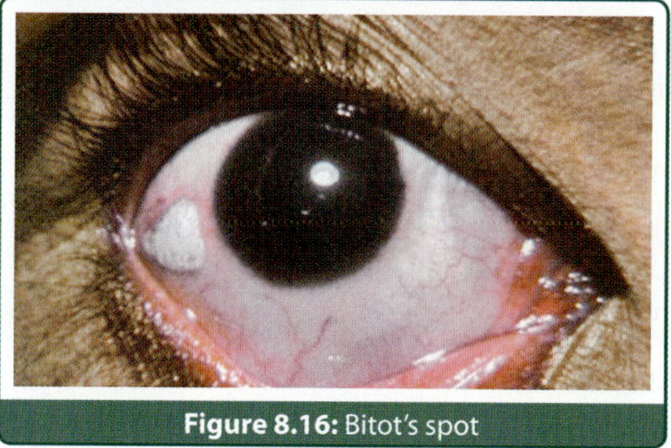

Figure 8.16: Bitot's spot

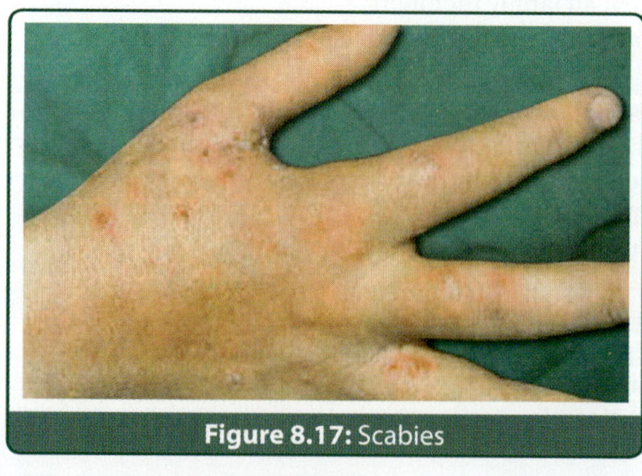

Figure 8.17: Scabies

5. **Turner's syndrome (Figs 8.18 to 8.20):**

Features of Turner's syndrome:

Gross appearance:
- Short stature
- Redundant nuchal skin (in utero cystic hygroma)
- Low posterior hairline
- Widespread nipples
- Shield chest
- Congenital lymphedema

Orthopedic:
- Patella dislocation
- Increased carrying angle of elbow (cubitus valgus)
- Madelung deformity (chondrodysplasia of distal radial epiphysis)
- Congenital hip dislocation
- Scoliosis

Cardiovascular system:
- Coarctation of aorta
- Bicuspid aortic valve
- Cardiac conduction abnormalities
- Hypoplastic left heart syndrome

ENT and Ophthal:
- Strabismus
- Cataracts
- Red-green color blindness (as in males)
- Recurrent otitis media
- Sensorineural hearing loss

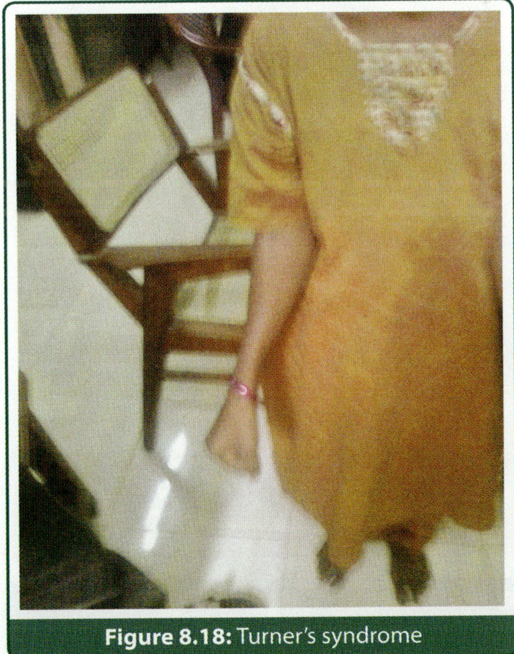

Figure 8.18: Turner's syndrome

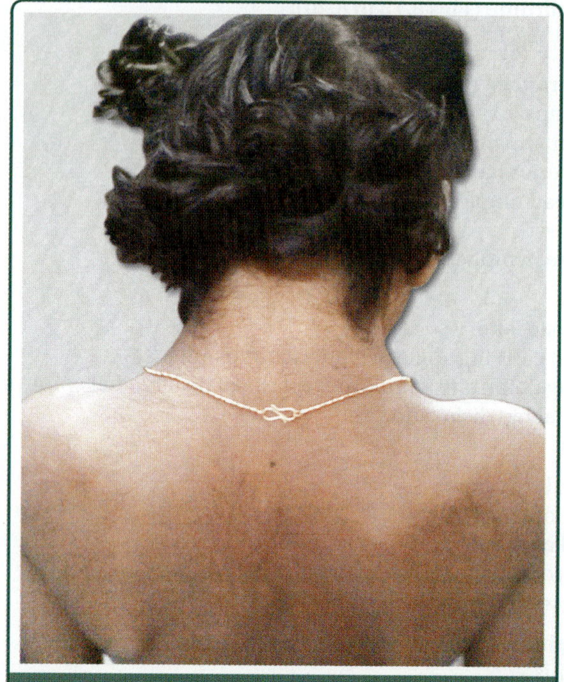

Figure 8.19: Turner's syndrome (Short neck)

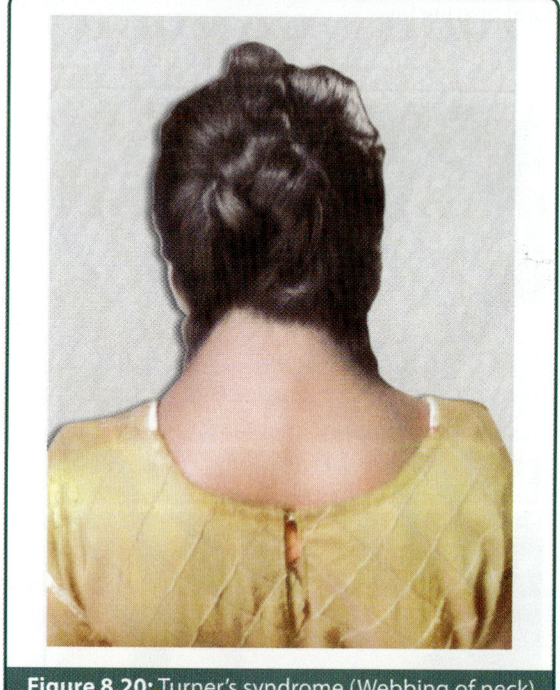

Figure 8.20: Turner's syndrome (Webbing of neck)

Reproductive:
- Gonadal dysgenesis (infertility, primary amenorrhea)
- Gonadoblastoma (increased risk if Y chromosome material is present)

Renal:
- Horseshoe kidneys

CNS:
- Learning disabilities (in 70%)
- Developmental delay (in 10%)
- Social awkwardness

Endocrine:
- Hypothyroidism (acquired in 15–30%)
- Type 2 diabetes mellitus (insulin resistance)

GIT:
- Inflammatory bowel disease
- Celiac disease (increased incidence)

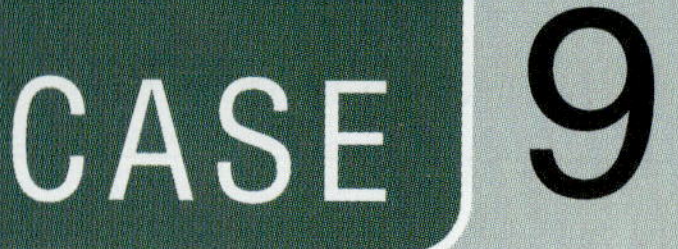

Vaccination

Vaccination: It Is the process of administering vaccines.
Immunization: It is the process of inducing immunity in host.

IMMUNITY

Active

Formed in the body following natural infection.

Passive

Formed antibody in the form of immunoglobulin (prepared outside).

Killed inactivated vaccines		*Live attenuated vaccines*	
Bacterial	***Viral***	***Bacterial***	***Viral***
Typhoid (whole cell) Cholera Pertussis	Salk(IPV) Hepatitis B subunit Rabies Influenza Japanese encephalitis	BCG Typhoid (oral) Plague	Oral polio vaccine Measles Mumps (MMR) Rubella Varicella

Expanded program on immunization (EPI) - started at 1973
Universal immunization programs (UIP) - started at 1985
In 1978 -Small pox Eradication

UNIVERSAL IMMUNIZATION PROGRAM (UIP)

- Birth : BCG, OPV0
- 6th week : DPT1, OPV1,
- 10th week : DPT2, OPV2
- 14th week: DPT3, OPV3
- 9 month: Measles
- 15–18 months: DPT and OPV, (booster 1)
- 5 years: DT
- 10 years: TT
- 16 years: TT

IAP Immunization Table 2011

Age	*Vaccines*
At birth	BCG OPV-0 HepB1
6 weeks	DTP1 OPV1/ OPV1+ IPV1 Hib1 HepB2 Rotavirus 1 PCV1
10 weeks	DTP2 OPV2/OPV2 + IPV2 Hib 2 Rotavirus2 PCV2
14 weeks	DTP3 OPV3/OPV3 + IPV3 Hib 3 Hep B3# Rotavirus3 PCV3
9th month	Measles
12th month	HepA1
15th month	MMR1 Varicella PCV Booster
16-18 months	DTP-Booster1 OPV4/OPV4 + IPV Booster1 *H influenzae* Booster1
2 years	Typhoid1
5 years	DTP-Booster2 OPV5 MMR2 Typhoid2 Varicella2*
10–12 years	Tetanus+ Diphtheria (Td)/Tdap HPV- Human papilloma virus vaccine only for females at 0, 1–2, 6 months

#- HepB- Third dose is given at 6th month
*- Varicella 2nd dose may be given at anytime, 3 months after 1st dose
=- Typhoid revaccination at every 3 years

IAP Immunization Table 2012

Age→ Vaccine↓	Birth	6 weeks	10 weeks	14 weeks	18 weeks	6 months	9 months	12 months	15 months	18 months	2–3 years	4–6 years
BCG	BCG											
HepB	HepB1	HepB2				HepB3						
Polio	OPV0	IPV1	IPV2	IPV3		OPV1	OPV2	IPVB1				OPV3
DTP		DTP1	DTP2	DTP3					DTPB1			DTPB2
Hib		Hib1	Hib2	Hib3				Hib-booster				
Pneumococcal		PCV1	PCV2	PCV3				PCV-booster			PPSV	
Rotavirus		RV1	RV2	RV^{+}3								
Measles							Measles					
MMR								MMR1				MMR2
Varicella									Varicella1			Varicella2
HepA								HepA1			HepA2	
Typhoid											Typhoid	
Influenza						Influenza (yearly)						
Meningococcal											Meningococcal	
Cholera								Cholera1 and 2				
Japanese encephalitis							JE					

Cold chain: Maintaining the recommended temperature from the site of manufacture to administration.

Reverse cold chain: The stool samples in acute flaccid paralysis (AFP) are maintained in the same temperature until it reaches the laboratory.

Herd immunity: It is the immunity in the community.

Freezer	*Only oral polio vaccine*
Uppermost compartment	BCG Measles
2nd compartment	HepB DPT DT TT
Lower most compartment	Diluents (normal saline)

Eradication criteria	*Elimination criteria*
1. No polio virus cases for 3 years	1. Absent career for 1 year
2. No mild virus in the community	2. Low temp is required for virus
3. Strict clinical and virological surveillance	

DISCUSSION OF IMPORTANT VACCINES

BCG Vaccine

- Strain: Prepared from attenuating virulent strain of *Mycobacterium bovis.* After 230 social subcultures, they were able to evolve a strain known as Bacille Calmette-Guérin
- At present, Danish 133 strain is used in production of BCG in Guindy, Chennai, India
- Live attenuated vaccine.

  Administration:
  0.05 mL (in newborn)
  - 1.1 mL (in others)
  - 0.05 mL contains 0.4 to 0.5 million bacilli
- Intradermally at the level of insertion of deltoid in the left arm

  Ideally given after birth. Why?
  - CMI (cell-mediated immunity) not transferred from mother
  - Endemicity
  - Low immunity in the body may go for disseminated TB, meningitis
- If the vaccine injected subcutaneously → abscess formation occurs

  Types of BCG:
  - Liquid (fresh)
  - Freeze-dried (more stable)

  Dosage bottle:
  - Each vial contains—10 doses (0.05 mL, 10 doses) in powder form

- Dilute with 2 mL **normal saline**
- Size of needle: 26 G
- Color of bottle: Ambe/Brown color to prevent exposure to sunlight.
- Reconstituted vaccine must be used in 3–4 hours. If not:
  i. Potency is lost
  ii. It is a live vaccine and there is no antibacterial substance, hence, easy contamination occurs.

Why should it be given in left shoulder?

1. Uniformity throughout
2. If given too above—cervical adenitis
   Too below—axillary adenitis

Protection:

i. Protects against severe form of TB (meningeal and disseminated TB)
ii. Used as therapeutic, diagnostic
iii. No protection against other diseases
iv. Used in cancer bladder treatment as immunotherapy

Reaction on administration:

- Immediately after intradermal injection 'Peau d'orange' elevation upto 5–8 mm occurs which confirms our injection is correctly intradermal
- It is a CMI, so the immunity develops after 3 weeks
  - After 4 weeks: Papule
  - After 5 weeks: Nodule
  - After 6 weeks: Ulcerates and heals alternatively
  - After 8 weeks: Scar

  If no scar formed after 12 weeks, repeat BCG.

Adverse Effects

- Regional adenitis (axillary, cervical nodes)
- Severe ulceration
- Local abscess—Rx: Aspiration, INH powder.

Contraindications: Immunodeficient individuals

Oral Polio Vaccine (OPV)

- Strain: Live attenuated virus (Type 1, 2, 3) grown in monkey kidney agar or HDC (human diploid cell)
- Tissue culture infective dose (TC id)- 10^6, $10^{5.5}$, 10^5 (of type 1, 2, 3)
- Stored in freezer
- Dosage bottle: Light pink vaccine—is due to addition of magnesium chlorate gives light pink color (stabilizing substance is Mg chlorate).

Administration

Tilt the child back, squeeze the cheeks to open the mouth. Let the drop falls from dropler into child's tongue.

- Two drops per dose
- Avoid breastfeeding before and after 15–30 minutes.

Why is it given immediately after birth?

- Colostrum helps in take up of the vaccine (Better give it before delivery of shoulder)
- Intestine clean: No interference in uptake.

Why should you give five such many doses?

1. Herd immunity
2. Take up of the vaccine is low
3. Vaccination failure

Vaccine vial monitor (VVM)
If the square inside matches the color outside becomes deeper discard.

Keep in freezer
Pulse Polio Vaccination—1995:
Two rounds, Booth based

- Given on public holidays (3rd Sunday of December and 3rd Sunday of January)
- To eliminate the polio
- **Why given on Oct/Nov/Dec?**
  - Load of units is low
  - Low temperature is required for vaccine virus.

Intensified polio (PPV)—1997

- Oct 1999- Jan 2000 (4 weeks - part)
- Each around for 3 days
- Day—post (Booth) Passed
- II/III days—house to house reach.

Surveillance for Acute Flaccid Paralysis (AFP)

Acute flaccid paralysis is defined as the acute onset of weakness of <4 weeks duration manifested as hypotonia, areflexia, flaccidity in 1 or 2 limbs

Differential diagnosis of AFP:

- Traumatic neuritis
- Transverse myelitis
- Poliomyelitis
- Guillain-Barré syndrome.

Contraindications for OPV

1. Acute infectious disease
2. Fever
3. Diarrhea
4. Dysentery

May not be given for:

1. Leukemia
2. Malignancy
3. Steroids

DPT

Administration

- 0.5 mL Intramuscular anterolateral aspect of thigh(or)
- Right side on deltoid
  - Not to inject in gluteal region—because due to increased fat, there will be low absorption and it is less immunogenic
- 0.5 mL contains:
  - 20 Loeffler units of diphtheria
  - 5 Loeffler units of tetanus
  - 4 IU of pertussis.

Killed vaccine

Why given at 6th/10th/14th week?

For convenience sake.

(Mother has to come for postnatal visit 6th, 10th and 14th week so we do both at same time;

Adverse effects:

- Inconsolable cry for >3 hours
- Hypotonic hyporesponsive episode <48 hours
- Fever >40.5°C/105°F
- Shock
- Convulsions (primary febrile convulsions)
- Acute encephalopathy (in 7 days)
- Seizures within 3 days

Avoid Pertussis in next dose and give DT alone

Contraindications

1. Progressive neurological disorder (DT can be used)
2. Cerebral palsy/fertile convulsions are not contraindications
3. Severe reaction to previous dose and prolonged cry.

Adults: Given DT

Measles

Strain: Live attenuated Edmonston Zagreb strain (name of the child from whom vaccine is derived)

Others: Moraten
Schwartz

Administration

- Subcutaneously 0.5 over right deltoid
- Used within 1-4 hours after opening
- Diluent is distilled water.

Why not given before 6 months?

- Residual maternal antibodies in the serum neutralizes the immunogenic property of vaccine.

Contraindications

- Malignancy and immunosuppression
- Antimetabolites
- Alkylating agents
- Corticosteroids
- Active TB (but can be given in HIV).

Adverse effect:

- Staphylococcal shock syndrome (SSS)
- Measles like illness—rash, arthralgia, fever.

Recent: Aerosol administration of measles may be (HDC preparation): Given at 4-6 months.

MMR: Live

- Strain: Measles—E-Z strain (Moraten, Schwartz)
- Mumps: Jeryl lynn strain
- Rubella: HPV 77/cendenhill/ RA(27/3)
  (Three strains of rubella).

Administration

0.5 mL SC over right deltoid.

Importance

- Rubella must be given to all female children
- Pre-pubertal immunization necessary.

Contraindication

Immunosuppression and pregnancy.

HIV and Vaccination
Asymptomatic HIV – BCG can be given
Symptomatic HIV – Avoid BCG/OPV/Varicella
Can give – DPT, MMR, IPV, HepB

Quick Reckoner

Vaccine	*Nature*	*Diluent*	*Storage*	*Dose*	*Route*	*Protective efficacy*
BCG	Live attenuated	**Normal saline**	Freezer/ 2–8°C	0.1 mL	Left deltoid **Intradermal**	0–80%
OPV	Live attenuated	Liquid vaccine	Freezer/ 2–8°C	2 drops	Oral	10–15% per dose
IPV	Inactivated	Liquid vaccine	2–8°C	0.5 mL	IM/SC thigh/ deltoid	95–100%
DTP		Liquid vaccine	2–8°C	0.5 mL	IM thigh/ deltoid	95–100 for diphtheria and tetanus 70–90% for pertussis

Contd...

Contd...

Vaccine	*Nature*	*Diluent*	*Storage*	*Dose*	*Route*	*Protective efficacy*
DT		Liquid vaccine	2–8°C	0.5 mL	IM Thigh/ deltoid	
Measles	Live attenuated	**Sterile water**	Freezer 2–8°C	0.5 mL	**SC** Thigh/ deltoid	80%
Rubella	Live attenuated	Sterile water	Freezer 2–8°C	0.5 mL	SC Thigh/ deltoid	95%
MMR	Live attenuated	Sterile water	Freezer 2–8°C	0.5 mL	SC Thigh/ deltoid	95%
HepB		Liquid vaccine	2–8°C	0.5 mL for <18 years and 1 mL for >18 years	IM Deltoid/ thigh	90%
H influenza B		Liquid vaccine Or Lyophilized that is diluted with sterile water	2–8°C	0.5 mL	IM Thigh/ deltoid 6,10,14 weeks Booster at 15–18 months	90%

Index

D

E

F

G

N

O

P

S

T